Successfully Coping With Fibromyalgia

The Chemical Triggers of Pain

Bruce Nelson

VI. A WORD.

A WORD is dead
When it is said,
Some say.
I say it just
Begins to live
That day.

Emily Dickinson, "Poems Series Three"
edited by Mabel Loomis Todd

Contents

Introduction 7
   How this book is organized 15
What's New 17
What is Fibromyalgia? 19
   Chapter Summary 26
My Fibromyalgia 27
   FM Pain 28
   Triggers 29
   Compounding Factors 30
   Compensations 30
   An FM Event 31
   The Fibromyalgia Balance 34
   The Symptoms of an FM Event 37
   Anatomy of a Pain Event 46
   Chapter Summary 49
Why is this Happening? 50
Triggers 56
   Figure 1: Fibromyalgia Trigger Factors 60
   Chemical Trigger: Yellow 6 61
   Trigger: Chocolate 67
   Chemical Trigger: Sodium Nitrate/Nitrite 71
   Chemical Trigger: Road Salt 76
   Trigger: Recovery from Illness/Lack of Sleep 88
   Chemical Trigger: Root Beer 90
   Chemical Trigger: Earl Grey Tea 92
   Additional Suspected Triggers 93
   Chapter Summary 98
Compounding Factors: 99
   Figure 2: Compounding Factors 101
   High Atmospheric Pressure 102

Mental Stress..102
Cold Weather..105
Lack of Restful Sleep 108
Daylight Saving Time 108
Undue Physical Stress................................109
Poor Posture 109
Chapter Summary 112

Compensations 113

Figure 3: Compensations 120
Compensations before FM symptoms appear:........121
Getting restful sleep..................................121
Avoiding trigger factors 126
Maintaining FM situational awareness 126
Managing stress 128
Exercise and posture..................................128
Compensations after FM symptoms appear: 133
Managing an approaching FM event......................133
Figure 4: Managing an Approaching Event 135
"Precursor" symptoms 135
Illustration 1: Trapezius Spasm Points 137
TENS - Transcutaneous electrical nerve stimulation 141
Illustration 2: TENS Pad Placement 145
Recovering from an FM event:....................146
Caffeine..147
Chapter Summary 149

Approach..150

Illustration 3: Hierarchy of Coping Actions....................152
Chapter Summary 159

Chemical Safety.................................... 160

Conclusions 163

Resources 170

Introduction

I feel obligated to begin this book with some caveats: this is not a technical manual, I am not trained in any medical field, nor am I an expert in chronic pain, fibromyalgia, or any other related syndrome. I do not work in a medical or related field and have no credentials to make claims that concern them. I have nothing to sell, and I do not explicitly endorse any products or services of any kind. This book is not intended as a diagnostic aid – if you think you have unexplained, chronic pain you need to consult a doctor for expert advice. I have no new scientific theories as to the physical origins of fibromyalgia.

Instead, this is a book about the success I've had in greatly reducing the degree and frequency of the painful events that once ruled my life – the chronic pain that I experience and my unique perspective as a sufferer. Admittedly, I'm a population of one individual but with many thousands of "samples" – the various events I've experienced over the years and the net results of trial and error in trying to prevent them and reduce their impact.

This is the second book I've written on this topic. Over ten years have passed since I released the book "Coping with Fibromyalgia", my first attempt to share what I had learned about many years of dealing with its pain and disruption. At that time, I felt I had learned as much as I was going to know about avoiding and managing its impacts, but I was wrong. I continued to expand on my original understanding and improved greatly over the intervening years, finding new ways to deal with and avoid the pain it brings.

The goal of this book is not to repeat the story I've related in "Coping with Fibromyalgia" but to expand on that earlier book and describe what I've learned since then. I refer you to that book for greater detail on my earlier experiences. While it is heavier on the path I took to awakening, this new one describes where I am today – miles ahead of where I began.

I've continued to practice the steps I had outlined in the earlier book and found new ways of responding to FM pain events as well as confirming what I already knew about triggers and taking steps to avoid and react to them. My success has been significant enough to require an update – both in content and in the title – moving from "Coping with Fibromyalgia" to "*Successfully* Coping with Fibromyalgia".

I've also had success by thinking more broadly about pain than the narrow definition of Fibromyalgia, though that was the original diagnosis I was given. I see that reflected in the research and assistance resources I have used in these past ten years – a widening of attention to chronic pain rather than its categorization into narrow specialties. In this volume, I'll continue to use the more specific term fibromyalgia, despite it falling out of favor. Regardless of what we call our version of chronic pain, I relate to the symptoms and feelings that are shared by a broader group than fibromyalgia covers, as well as many of the core actions taken to alleviate them.

Unfortunately, we have seen no breakthrough in the treatment of the symptoms that affect so many people around the world. The current opioid crisis demonstrates just how desperate the need is for pain abatement, and the lack of safe, direct treatment alternatives. Yes, we have seen a growing awareness of the disease (or condition or syndrome) under the term "chronic pain" over that same time, and an acceptance from the medical community that it's real – more than the psychological condition it was once felt to be. Yet there is no silver bullet, no magic substance that will negate this special kind of pain, not rooted in disease or inflammation but arising unexpectedly and failing to respond to traditional measures.

I've now reached a point where pain is the rare exception rather than a constant, underlying reality, and where I have an explanation for each event I experience. While everything I had said in the first edition remains true, my experience since then has served to turn those recommendations on their head – to favor avoidance over treatment.

It is now clear to me that avoidance is possible in almost all cases – I can trace a pain event back to its source and find ways to prevent it by avoiding (or mitigating) exposure to a triggering substance. In the rare case where avoidance isn't possible or practical, all the mitigating "compensations" I had identified remain true and useful to reduce or overcome the pain. But I rarely need them now – I've found the source of almost every FM pain event and, so long as I avoid these triggering factors, I'm free of pain.

Even in the early days of dealing with FM events (the 1980s), I was suspicious that each event had a cause that, if identified, could be avoided rather than treated. Not as a cure that treated the pain itself, but as a behavioral change that would prevent its occurrence in the first place. At that early date, some causes (such as a certain yellow dye – yellow 6) were very clear - exposure to any amount of that substance predictably resulted in FM pain – but I continued to experience events I couldn't explain and so continued to focus first on pain management. Much of the first edition was devoted to that end – managing pain. In this new volume, I'm bringing the focus back to the techniques I use to avoid pain events in the first place.

In short – this book reflects these new learnings by emphasizing avoidance of the triggering factors I now realize are needed for me to experience FM pain. Compensating for the resulting pain now takes a back seat to avoiding it altogether. Avoidance of environmental factors leads me directly to a life without FM pain for extended periods. I can now honestly say I am successfully coping with the chronic pain of fibromyalgia.

One final explanation – much of the content of this new volume is, of necessity, a restatement of the earlier "Coping with Fibromyalgia". It is necessary to set the stage in the same manner as before, but almost every aspect of the earlier book has been amended, either to confirm the original findings or expand them with new detail. I've found several new triggers and substantial new compensations that I need to share, along with the original material.

Read my earlier book "Coping with Fibromyalgia" for a more detailed account of how I reached the stage where I felt that I had fibromyalgia under control. Yet I continued to make progress in managing pain, on both sides of events. I've learned of new substances that trigger events and new ways to deal with pain when avoidance fails. It's an evolving process – perhaps I can return in another ten years or so to report a "cure".

So, twelve years later and I've turned this story around completely – I now focus on the behavioral changes needed to avoid pain events rather than on the steps needed to compensate for them. It turns the original book on its head – I now focus on the avoidance of triggers (in the Factors and Approach chapters), rather than treating symptoms (in the Compensations chapter). So long as I maintain good health and avoid the substances that trigger fibromyalgia in my body – I'm fine. I'm seeing very few "FM events". Even if I fail, I have new ways to cope that are far more successful and less invasive than in the past.

It's now clear that I have a good handle on the factors that trigger FM in me – and I was correct in my assumption that it was largely substances I encounter in food and the environment. If I avoid these chemicals I'm fine – exposure leads to an FM event. It remains true that certain things increase my susceptibility, but I'm now convinced that a triggering substance is needed in almost all cases before I'll experience FM pain.

I'll expand on all this in the sections that follow, but in some sense this *is* the end of the story I was looking for. I've found ways to prevent FM pain for long periods (weeks or months at a time) and know why it occurs in the rare instances that I now experience it. I can anticipate its arrival and take measures to head it off. When I do see FM pain it's at a much lower level than in the past, and I have new compensating actions work much better to mitigate the pain.

~

And yet - I can still fall into symptoms of FM. I'm not "cured" in the sense that many modern treatments might promise. My symptoms are lessened, but not completely absent. A pill wasn't enough to affect a cure – to complete the treatment and banish FM symptoms forever – and that's where this book begins. It's still necessary for me to pay strict attention to my behavior, what I eat, what substances I might be exposed to, how well I sleep, my posture, how much and what type of exercise I get, and more. All this is needed to reduce the symptoms beyond the initial relief afforded by the avoidance and compensation techniques I've learned. Without these behaviors and activities, I quickly fall back into pain. I would still term this "coping with" rather than "curing" my underlying fibromyalgia.

There must be other modern maladies that follow this same pattern – where a pill will not be enough for a complete cure, where behavioral change is needed to complete the treatment working along with the traditional medical approaches. I also suspect that systemic and regulatory changes in managing the food chain and our environment are needed to reduce our exposure to a variety of substances that are the cause of undesirable side effects.

Finally – and importantly – I am using the term "coping" here in a broader sense than its formal definition suggests. It's the 21st-century notion, meaning both the identification of potential stressful problems and events and the active measures intended to resolve them. This is "Active" rather than "Passive" coping – including measures I can take to avoid or mitigate stressful pain events rather than simply enduring them, as in the past.

I'll go into greater detail on all this in later chapters where I will describe all the measures that work for me to manage my symptoms – to actively cope. I will describe actions that work for me to reduce FM to a manageable level, to a point where I feel I am luckier than most normal people in the quality of life I can achieve.

How this book is organized

What's New outlines the changes this book presents over my original book "Coping with Fibromyalgia", written in 2001 and due for an update with new information I've learned in the intervening years.

What is Fibromyalgia? is an overview of fibromyalgia as I see it today, in 2023.

My Fibromyalgia is a description of how I experience the pain and other symptoms of this condition, as well as how I've come to view it. I define the terms I use throughout the rest of the book, some of which are unique to my understanding of what I'm experiencing.

Why is this Happening? is my view of how we have reached a point where large numbers of people suffer pain with no specific diagnosis or hope for a cure, as well as my speculation as to at least one cause: the chemical triggers of pain.

In the **Triggers** chapter I describe each of the chemical and physical triggers that I have found to be a cause of pain, their impact on me and how I deal with them.

Compounding Factors outlines factors I see contributing to the onset and degree of pain.

Compensations covers general actions I take to prevent or reduce pain events beyond those I take to address specific triggers.

Approach describes how I cope with the day-to-day challenges presented to me by fibromyalgia, and how these might relate to others with this condition. It's the practical effect of what I've covered in the prior chapters, describing how I live my life given the chemical triggers of pain I contact in my environment.

Chemical Safety is a short observation as to how difficult it is to find unbiased, complete information on the modern chemicals to which we are exposed daily.

Conclusions is a short summary of this entire book – my statement as to what I'm facing and why I seem to be alone in reporting it. It includes the actions I believe are needed to address the chemical triggers of pain.

Resources lists the sources I've used to learn more about fibromyalgia and the chemicals that trigger it in my body, as well as the measures I've learned to take when dealing with it.

What's New

Here is a quick list of the major updates over the original "Coping with Fibromyalgia". The earlier book remains valid but reflects a different state of awareness than I now have today. It goes into much greater detail on how my awareness of fibromyalgia began and evolved, describing how I managed FM pain in 2011, but it's not telling the full story.

This volume reflects major new findings and the progress I've made in managing FM pain over the intervening twelve years. It starts where I left off in 2011 and describes how my view of managing fibromyalgia has evolved since then. This new thinking includes:

A new, clearer understanding of the triggers behind my pain that turns my view of its causes on its head. This includes newly identified "triggers" – chemicals in my food and the environment that directly trigger symptoms, factors I only found in the intervening years between these volumes. It also reflects my realization that a trigger is always needed before I experience FM pain, and that it's almost always a chemical one.

A major new technique for warding off the progression of pain into a full-blown "FM Event". I'm able to use a TENS device (transcutaneous electric nerve stimulation) to significantly reduce the impact of fibromyalgia in my life.

Better awareness of the progression of events leading up to pain and new ways to compensate for each of the various triggers behind it.

My guess as to what is really behind my experience with chronic pain. I refuse to believe I'm alone in my unique physical world, others must be affected similarly. I'll also explain how I think we got here – with no noteworthy progress over the forty-plus years I've been afflicted with unexplained, chronic pain.

While this may seem like a brief list of changes, they have resulted in a revision of every section of the original volume to reflect the acceptance of environmental causes for nearly every FM Event I experience.

Combined, these greatly increase my ability to "successfully cope" with fibromyalgia beyond the improvements I was able to report in 2011.

What is Fibromyalgia?

Here in early 2023 Fibromyalgia is defined on the Mayo Clinic website as ... "a disorder characterized by widespread musculoskeletal pain accompanied by fatigue, sleep, memory, and mood issues". A lengthy list of associated symptoms is shown across the various medical sources that describe this condition. Wikipedia's suggested diagnosis is based on the presence of symptoms "after ruling out other potential causes".

As to the underlying cause, the consensus today – in early 2023 - from all the official and unofficial sources I've come to rely on over the years remains a resounding "we don't know". That's my summary of the current definition of fibromyalgia as it appears in Wikipedia, the respected internet source I've come to trust as a great place to start when looking for information on a new subject. It's seconded in the many health sites available on the internet devoted to fibromyalgia including the Mayo Clinic, WebMD, and others.

To begin, let's get some terms defined as their use in describing fibromyalgia has changed over the years. Here's my summary from multiple sources:

A **disease** is a pathophysiological response to internal or external factors.

A **disorder** is a disruption to regular bodily structure and function.

A **syndrome** is a collection of signs and symptoms associated with a specific health-related cause.

A **condition** is an abnormal state of health that interferes with normal or regular feelings of well-being.

Health sources today – in 2023 – most often describe fibromyalgia as a "condition" rather than a syndrome, I suspect due to the continuing inability to identify a specific physiological cause. The term "syndrome" was popular when I wrote "Coping with Fibromyalgia" in 2011 but it no longer seems to be in widespread use.

It's not considered a "disease" or "disorder". While there is agreement that something bad is going on, there is no scientific consensus as to the underlying cause for these symptoms.

No, that's not a satisfactory answer. Yet it's all we have given the current state of research and medical investigation. At this point, there isn't even complete agreement that the symptoms currently being described as "fibromyalgia" are, in fact, a syndrome - let alone what the underlying cause may be.

In comparison, migraine is considered a syndrome though there seems to be some agreement as to its classification as a disease. Fibromyalgia is earlier in the scientific discovery cycle and there seems to be greater disagreement about its status.

To give some idea of the lack of progress we've seen I performed a modest test: I compared the Mayo Clinic website page describing Fibromyalgia between October 2007 to December 2022. (See the appendix for links, but it's possible to access snapshots of web pages taken at specific points in the past and saved for historical purposes by using the Archive.org "Wayback Machine").

I won't replicate them here, but the two snapshots are nearly identical (some minor rewording has taken place), except for diagnosis – where the "tender point exam" of the past has been replaced by reported pain in four of five "areas". They have also added a need for additional testing to be sure you aren't suffering from a known disease.

The Mayo Clinic diagnosis tends to be more specific than any other classification criteria – the current Wikipedia page lists around ten various techniques, stating that the criteria have evolved over time.

My summary of the current methods of diagnosis is "widespread pain for three or more months with no other diagnosable disorder present". A host of other symptoms may be present but are not universally required for a diagnosis of fibromyalgia. Pain seems to be the predominant symptom, pain that is not otherwise explained by a different underlying disease. The "associated symptoms" form such a wide range of experiences I'm reluctant to try and list them all.

Fibromyalgia has recently been described by one researcher as a "bitterly controversial condition", its existence as a diagnosis remains questioned in some medical circles. (For a relatively recent overview see "Facts and myths pertaining to fibromyalgia", Winfried Häuser, MD and Mary-Ann Fitzcharles, MD " – there's a link in the resources section).

Essentially, a diagnosis of fibromyalgia only means you have reached an agreement with a member of the medical profession that the constellation of signs and symptoms you are reporting does not match any other known illness – based on the objective measures known to science and used widely for diagnosing disease –

and that they correlate with (generally match) those that have become accepted as the syndrome currently called "fibromyalgia". There are no laboratory tests that prove the presence of fibromyalgia – a diagnosis is made based on the symptoms experienced – though tests may be needed to rule out other disorders.

A quick aside – it's important to rule out diseases for which we have solutions. If you experience chronic pain, you need medical assistance to reach this conclusion. That's something of which we *are* capable.

In terms of demographics the U.S. Centers for Disease Control and Prevention reports that fibromyalgia afflicts about four million Americans, but the American College of Rheumatology estimates 2-4% of the population (that would be 7 to 14 million Americans as of December 2022). If this incidence can be applied worldwide (and that's a big if) there may be 160 to 320 million people with fibromyalgia worldwide.

It was once seen as primarily affecting women (where it was once thought that as many as 90% of sufferers were female) but figures now suggest it afflicts twice as many women as men (that would be 33% men, 66% women).

The current Wikipedia article for Fibromyalgia doesn't even list a heading for "Treatment", but instead uses the term "Management", citing a recent professional review article in "Current Rheumatology Reports" that states *There is no definitive cure for fibromyalgia and treatment primarily focuses on both symptom management and improving patient quality of life.* "

I should point out that I've never met the full criteria as defined in the Mayo Clinic guide. I don't experience tender points below the waist and my pain is normally found primarily on one side of my upper body at any one time.

While I can relate to almost the full constellation of signs and symptoms described above to a certain extent, for me the primary issue is pain. It's an unusual kind of pain – not your normal pain of a pulled muscle, cut, or injury. It's accompanied by fatigue, but pain is the primary symptom with fatigue only appearing with the most significant events. Over-the-counter pain relievers provide no effective relief.

I should also point out the similarities I see between my symptoms and those of migraine. I experience visual migraines – though not in conjunction with pain. They occur all on their own, without pain, and not necessarily in association with fibromyalgia symptoms. I can also relate to the phases of migraine – the lead-up to pain, the pain itself, and to a certain extent the post-pain phase. And yet I rarely experience headache pain – my pain is better described by the body aches, muscle spasms, and sensitive spots once called fibromyalgia.

I also see parallels between my own fibromyalgia "triggers" and those reported by migraine sufferers, as well as in the way certain factors influence susceptibility. It seems likely we may share an approach to dealing with the pain, as well. While I can only describe my own experience with fibromyalgia, I hope my unique approaches might help migraine sufferers as well.

All this is not to say that we know nothing about fibromyalgia and similar sources of chronic pain. I would strongly urge everyone having symptoms that fall into this category to read widely and continue reading, new insights appear regularly. For anyone wanting a more clinical and descriptive list of symptoms, I'll refer you to the "Resources" section of this book where I've listed many of the sources I've used over the years to better understand fibromyalgia.

Chapter Summary

- There is no consensus on the underlying cause of fibromyalgia within the broader category of "chronic pain".
- It is generally described as a "condition" or disorder - an abnormal state of health, though there's disagreement on any further details.
- There has been no progress on identifying an underlying cause.
- My summary of the current methods of diagnosis: widespread pain for three or more months with no underlying condition being diagnosed.
- "No other condition being diagnosed" is an important caveat - many known conditions may mimic its symptoms.
- As many as 320 million people worldwide may be afflicted.
- It may afflict twice as many women as men - though that's a major increase in men, once seen as a minor part of the total.
- There is no known cure, only treatments that manage the symptoms.

My Fibromyalgia

So far, I've restricted myself to the characterization of fibromyalgia by authoritative sources who largely limit themselves to a description of pain not otherwise explained by any known cause and to the various remedies available that treat the related symptoms.

It's time to turn this on its head – as the source of pain in my case is very clear to me – it is almost exclusively due to exposure to various modern chemicals in our food and the environment.

Nearly all the pain events I experience can be traced back to one of a relatively short list of substances that I'm in contact with. If I avoid exposure to them – I'm without pain. If I come into direct contact with them – I experience a pain event.

An event doesn't closely follow exposure – it's not as if I'm being poisoned – it's a gradual tip into pain that begins hours after exposure, as in 8 to 14 plus hours later, and extends for 12 to 24 hours or more after it begins.

The direct tie between trigger exposure and pain wasn't clear to me in 2011 when I wrote the original "Coping with Fibromyalgia" book. I hadn't found all the substances, nor had I been through enough pain events to confirm all that I suspected at the time. After many more iterations of exposure and pain, this pattern is clear. Exposure equals pain, avoidance equals normality.

My confidence in the clarity of this relationship resolves a lot of the uncertainty I reported in 2011 about what triggers a pain event.

~

In describing my approach to identifying and dealing with the causes of my FM events, I'm forced to invent my own terms to describe how I view it. I'll elaborate on each of these terms later in the book but first let me set the stage with a few brief formal definitions.

FM Pain

I won't need to reinvent the term pain here, but let me refine what I mean by it in FM terms:

FM pain isn't the acute pain of say, a broken bone or sprained ankle. It's not the recurrent or intermittent pain of a toothache. It doesn't match the symptoms of an allergic reaction or poisoning.

It's not accompanied by any visible damage: swelling or redness or warmth.

It is instead "chronic", or long term - at least it can reach that stage. For me, it has characteristics that overlap other types of pain, particularly in the early stages, but develops into a unique type that I recognize from long experience. It's pain, pure and simple (and disabling) accompanied by fatigue.

Triggers

I'm defining a trigger as something that directly causes my FM symptoms. Almost every pain event I experience can be traced back to a substance I ingest or I'm physically exposed to in some way. These clearly initiate pain and are the direct cause of an FM event and so I'll call them triggers. They somehow trigger pain in my body.

These triggers are not to be confused with FM "trigger points" – specific locations in the body that are related to pain. The triggers I'm describing here are almost all substances that I've come to believe trigger, or directly cause my FM symptoms. There are two exceptions to the rule that they are chemical in nature – lack of sleep and recovery from illness.

Compounding Factors

Compounding factors are things that can increase FM pain, but which generally do not result in an event without an actual trigger being experienced. I'm calling these compounding factors as they increase the likelihood of experiencing pain and its eventual severity should I be exposed to a trigger.

Compensations

Compensations are the actions I take to avoid an FM event or to deal with it once pain begins. I say actions because that best describes what it takes me to prevent FM symptoms from occurring. I've had only limited success with pharmacological solutions (medicine, herbs, or the like). Most of the actions that work for me would better be described as "techniques".

When I say compensation I'm using it in the full meaning of the term – it's not a cure, it's a set of actions, behaviors, and thought patterns that tend to reduce the severity of symptoms. When I experience symptoms, I'm able to reduce them significantly in severity and duration. I'm even able to forestall the appearance of a full-blown "FM Event".

Some compensations are specific to their trigger, others are more general in nature.

An FM Event

I am defining an "FM event" as the progression of pain and other FM symptoms over time, from initiation to relief. These include a plateau of symptoms that are life-disrupting and undesirable. For me, these are primarily expressed as widespread pain and fatigue, though other sufferers report a broader array of symptoms. While I can relate to these other symptoms and experience many of them, pain and fatigue are my primary complaints. Managing this pain seems to bring relief from all the other symptoms I associate with fibromyalgia.

At its worst (I'll call this a "full-blown" event), an FM event can literally knock me to the floor. It's a unique kind of pain that defies comparison to anything else I've ever experienced. It often begins with a dull pressure and tightness in my shoulder, neck, and back muscles. It can vary in the muscle groups it involves and in severity, it can move around over time, but it always has the potential to become overwhelming. I can usually fight it off for a time, putting up a brave front and ignoring the pain, but it catches up to me eventually when I'm no longer able to deny it, often in the late afternoon or evening after the day's activities or work have ended.

I see this as an event because it has a predictable progression of steps:

- **prolog** – exposure to a trigger (perhaps only identified later, after the symptoms begin).
- **onset** - when symptoms start to appear (some hours later).
- **buildup** – the progression of pain which, without intervention, can become incapacitating.
- **crescendo** (maximum pain, perhaps extending for hours or even days).
- **release** (as symptoms slowly abate).
- **normality**, a return to my original, normal, pain and symptom-free state (albeit often weary).

I'll describe how I experience an FM event in greater detail at a later point, but this progression of symptoms is much clearer to me today having identified the major triggers at play and having found new ways to compensate for them.

~

With these definitions behind us let me start anew on the topic of triggers and compensations.

I'm separating these two aspects of coping with FM simply because I've found thinking about it in this way can be useful and successful. It is a technique that I have found to work in the daily effort to cope with its effects. Thinking in these terms can be a challenge at times, particularly when you are under the influence of the very pain you're trying to avoid, but I believe it has been one of the keys to my ability to find significant relief.

What I'm suggesting here isn't easy. Rather than focusing on the pain itself and the modern techniques and pharmacological solutions available to treat pain directly, focus instead on what you were doing before the advent of pain. What actions may have led up to pain? What were you doing or eating recently? What might the trigger behind the pain be?

I'm also suggesting you focus on what you may *not* have been doing before the pain, such as getting the right amount and kind of exercise, sleep, or nutrients in your diet.

What I'm *not* suggesting here is that you ignore pain management techniques and measures; I am suggesting instead that you focus primarily on avoidance, not amelioration. First: find and avoid pain triggers, second: take compensating actions. Consider the use of pain reduction measures as the failure of your active coping effort, as motivation to continue the effort to identify the root causes behind the pain and to redouble your efforts to avoid or otherwise ameliorate it. Make pain management the last tool in your war chest, not the first.

The Fibromyalgia Balance

Twelve years ago, in "Coping with Fibromyalgia" I described a process I termed "the fibromyalgia balance". Akin to walking a tightrope, I saw managing FM symptoms as a balancing act between normality and pain, with a host of factors providing a positive and negative boost to "susceptibility". Some actions and activities (including exposure to triggers) eventually led to an FM event, some helped fend it off. "Coping" was needed to maintain that balance and prevent an event from occurring.

In describing the factors that lead up to FM pain I once thought of them in two categories: those that tended to result in FM symptoms in and of themselves: trigger factors, and those that seemed to influence my susceptibility, making FM symptoms more likely to occur: susceptibility factors.

I now think about this in a somewhat different manner.

It's now clear to me that the balancing aspect of coping was an outgrowth of failing to manage all the triggers I'm exposed to. I only had some triggers identified and managed. This led to an ongoing, underlying level of pain that wasn't fully controlled. I was reducing – but not controlling – FM triggers.

Having found all the triggers I normally experience in my daily life I can honestly drop the "balancing" aspect and describe things in a far more black-and-white manner. If I'm exposed to certain chemicals in the environment, I experience pain. No chemical trigger exposure means no pain.

Admittedly – there may be triggers I have not yet found, substances I'm sensitive to but haven't encountered. This could be described as a balance of sorts between a carefully choreographed diet and physical environment and exposure to new triggers, but it's not the same balance as before.

I still see an underlying aspect of "susceptibility" as in how fast and easy a trigger can take effect and how much pain can result. Yet I'm consistently able to track back to a "trigger" – almost always a substance – that starts the pain in motion.

Now that I have a handle on the triggers that cause my FM symptoms, I've been able to move from a goal of reducing symptoms to avoiding them entirely. This has resulted in a very different experience, one that has become more predictable and less likely to result in a full-blown "FM event". I'm more often able to predict an upcoming pain event and take actions to reduce its impact, resulting in FM symptoms being expressed as an underlying predilection to pain rather than the certainty of a full event.

While I can't avoid triggers entirely (I would have to live a monkish life) I still experience pain, though much reduced due to new ways to compensate (more on that later). I can often manage it to a low level and continue with daily life.

For the sake of completeness let me describe what we're up against if those compensations aren't made or should they fail to work. The result: a full-blown "FM Event" in all its glory.

The Symptoms of an FM Event

A classic "FM event" for me is a progression that plays out over a period of hours or days rather than an "attack" that happens suddenly and unexpectedly. There is a progression of symptoms that lead up to pain, the arrival of pain itself, and then the subsidence of pain over a certain amount of time. Like a sine wave, the overall patterns of symptoms of an FM event follow a path of increasing severity until they reach their maximum point and then decrease until I reach relative normalcy again.

Let me describe the classic experience I would see before my new compensation techniques. I'll expand on the definitions I provided above, stage by stage:

Prolog

This is the initiation of an event - exposure to a trigger. I may know the trigger ahead of time (for example, with road salt) or exposure may be unexpected, hiding the prolog until the pain begins and requiring me to think back in an attempt to identify a potential trigger. It's not a "poisoning", it takes time for symptoms to appear – from 8 to 24 hours or longer. During this time, I feel completely normal.

Onset

Tension is often the first indication that something isn't quite right. The onset of pain begins with a characteristic feeling in my back and shoulders that is hard to describe, but one that I know well. Another indication can be pain in my face, a characteristic sign that my exposure to road salt hasn't been fully mitigated.

Hours have passed between the exposure to a trigger and the onset of pain. Some triggers are stronger and take effect sooner, others longer (for example, the nitrates in cured meat may take only 3 or 4 hours while road salt may take 8 to 12 or more hours).

Buildup

The tension and pain begin slowly, building gradually and spreading across my back and shoulders. It can also appear like increasing downward pressure in my upper body along with overall fatigue. It takes several hours for this to develop and may be deferred or stopped by the compensating actions I'll describe elsewhere.

I generally feel the onset of pain in certain characteristic areas in my back and shoulders, face, and neck. The focus moves around between these spots, but they are the same ones I've come to know from long experience.

Crescendo

This is the maximum extent of pain, often involving muscle knots and the corresponding acute pain that comes with them. Without compensating actions this could last for 8 to 24 hours or more and require me to retire to a dark room and lay on an exercise map covered by quilt to stay warm and quiet. It's also accompanied by fatigue, though I find it difficult to sleep while the pain is present. It's debilitating, overwhelming pain that can be deferred for a short time, but which must eventually progress to its full extent. I would describe it as a "multi-day long migraine".

I believe that most of the acute pain I experience comes with muscle spasms, rather than the trigger points that are present and uncomfortable, but less acutely painful. Some relief can come through manipulating these tender areas, but the pain itself is not centered in them.

In the past this simply had to be accepted and endured, there was nothing that reduced the intensity and duration of this phase of an FM event. That's not the case today, as I'll describe later in the Compensations section.

Release

Eventually, the pain will begin to ebb, and the muscle knots loosen, perhaps allowing me to sleep and begin to recover.

Normality

A return to a relatively pain-free life – most likely many hours after onset.

~

An important caveat: before I found and avoided most of the pain triggers I was in contact with, my fibromyalgia symptoms were characterized by an underlying level of constant pain – I was forever stuck in the onset and buildup phases. In the past these levels would overlap and leave me in constant (chronic) pain with multiple triggers in effect at any one point in time - making it difficult to identify the individual contributors.

This was what "normal" looked like to me as pain never abated – it was interrupted by intermittent bouts of more severe FM events that were disabling, but which never fully abated. I was able to defer the full-blown FM events into the evening and continue working, not knowing any better, but never fully recovering. It was only after I began to take remediation measures – early in my FM travels – that I realized just how much pain I had been in.

Having identified and controlled the environmental and diet triggers I found a new normal. I began to see the levels of pain more clearly: normality as the absence of pain; a level that's stuck in the onset/buildup phases with a nagging, but not debilitating amount of pain; and yet another level that continues through buildup, crescendo, and release – a full-blown event.

I'll describe specific triggers and their characteristics later – but some (for example, yellow dye and nitrates) tend to quickly break through into the FM event phase. Road salt tends to remain in the onset phase for extended periods, eventually developing into a full-blown FM event if I don't adequately compensate for it.

These days I'm seldom blind-sided by the onset of an event, as I would have been in the past. I'm able to anticipate its arrival knowing that I've been exposed to a trigger and predicting the outcome. I'm also better aware of the precursor symptoms – I've learned not to ignore them. Finally, by identifying and avoiding triggers I'm experiencing far fewer events overall (as in one every month or two, at most).

The two main exceptions to this success are chocolate and road salt. If I'm not careful with new sources/brands/types of chocolate I can experience a typically huge FM event – which I strongly suspect stems from a yellow dye being used to alter the color of the product. Road salt is an exception because it's not practical to avoid it entirely.

With the compensating techniques I've discovered in the past twelve years the incapacitation I previously saw is seldom reached. I continue to experience pain in the "onset" phase, but even there I have a new technique to short-circuit the pain. But more on this later.

For me, pain is the predominant symptom throughout an FM event, but is by no means the only one. Fatigue is often present, especially around the peak of pain. If the event is a strong one, I may also have a general feeling of unwellness, losing my appetite and interest in almost everything going on around me.

Unexplained FM events are now extremely rare and usually mean I should be looking for a recent food item that contains an unexpected or unlisted ingredient. I must think back to what I've eaten, or have been doing, that might have led to the event. It may not be the best time for analytical thinking but it's the best time to catch the factors that may have been potential causes - when the exposure is fresh in my mind.

At its height, an FM event can feel like I've pulled multiple muscles in my shoulders, neck, and back. The specific muscles that are affected can vary, but the nature of the pain is similar across events. The severity and length of the event can also vary – but at its worst can simply knock me to the floor in short order. At this elevated level, it is characterized by incapacitating, overwhelming and acute pain of a kind I've never experienced in any other way. Pain at 11 on a scale of 1 to 10 because, mercifully, you forget how bad it has been in the calmer periods between events.

Almost all the FM pain I experience comes above my waist, high in my chest, back, neck, and even in my face and jaw. It's an odd kind of pain with the burning, almost hot pain of numerous muscle spasms combined with an underlying general discomfort unique to FM. It's not the pain of an injury. I can clearly remember sliding on a hill in winter during my childhood, falling off my sled onto a rock. I can still recall the acute pain, could show you the very spot I landed, and perhaps even pick out the rock. I lay there on the frozen ground for a long time unable to move, nothing broken but in too much pain to stand. Eventually it subsided and I walked home.

But FM pain isn't like that for me – it builds more gradually, lasts longer at its peak, and tails off much more slowly. It becomes acute in a more overwhelming way, rather than as a point source of discomfort. It sometimes feels more like pressure or weight than pain, as if I were carrying a heavy, wet blanket over my shoulders while at the same time being in pain.

In addition to pain, sensitivity to sound and light characterizes my most serious FM events. Reducing these stimuli by resting in a dark and quiet room is a requirement for recovering from an event at this level of impact. Once I reach this stage, I need to find a way to disengage completely from further activity.

Fatigue is often associated with my FM events although it can be unclear whether it is the result of being in pain and perhaps sleeping poorly or if it's simply a part of FM itself.

While I can relate to many other reported FM symptoms it's the pain that I've come to define an FM event by – it's the first sign of an impending event, the one that's most impactful to my life and activities, the symptom that I have no quick fix for and the one I work hardest to avoid. I can only speak for myself in this – I realize that this pattern may not be the case for everyone who suffers with FM.

I should also point out that I have allergies (generally to pollen), but those symptoms are better described as allergic rhinitis, not including pain or fatigue, and are seldom associated in time with my FM events.

The end of the event can come quickly, or slowly. It may be gone the next morning or fade away on its own in a matter of a few minutes. It can come and go for several days. It can subside over a matter of several hours. It eventually becomes a memory only to be recovered with the onset of another FM event.

At the height of my FM susceptibility – more than 25 years ago now – I was in some sort of pain pretty much constantly. Today, knowing more about the substances that trigger FM events, I'm better able to avoid or moderate exposure. Without exposure to road salt, the spring, summer, and fall months are relatively pain-free. When I do experience an FM event, I now have ways to mitigate it that I didn't have in the past.

Anatomy of a Pain Event

Here's a timeline for a recent FM event I experienced when trying out a new chocolate product.

To set the stage, I was overconfident as I hadn't experienced a major FM event in months. My mistake was to try two items I wasn't sure of – a new chocolate and a new muffin. My diet was otherwise "safe", I was only eating foods I was sure of from experience.

I was trying this new chocolate as the brand was recommended by Consumer Reports magazine as having products low in cadmium and lead, two contaminants they were tracking in a variety of chocolate brands. (I later found this specific item was *not* low in either, but high in both, per the independent testing group "As You Sow").

Day 0	Noon	I try a new chocolate bar from a brand I've eaten before, but in a new "super dark" chocolate form. I limit myself to a single 1.5 oz piece. I know I'm taking a risk but hope for the best.
	9 PM	I go to bed, feeling normal.
Day 1	2 AM	I'm awakened by a characteristic pain in my mid-

		back, it's immediately apparent I've been exposed to a trigger of some kind. I begin to ask myself "what have I been doing recently?", having forgotten about the chocolate.
	3 AM	I realize this isn't going to pass and apply my TENS pads to my waist and start using it on my normal settings.
	8 AM	TENS is not helping this time – I begin to suspect the food dye "yellow 6" and remember I tried a new chocolate bar at lunch the previous day, along with a new English muffin containing hemp seeds. I haven't been exposed to road salt recently. It's now clear this is going to be a major FM event.
	All day and overnight	I remain in bed, napping and intermittently using the TENS unit – which only seems to take the edge off the pain, not block it entirely. (It's a help - I'm not driven to lie on the floor over an exercise mat, my "final solution" to a full-blown FM event.) The pain moves from one area to another on my back over the hours, accompanied by fatigue.
Day 2	9 AM	I'm finally able to rise and sit in a chair, watching television and

		intermittently using the TENS unit.
	7 PM	I retire and I'm able to sleep somewhat normally.
Day 3	--	As I recover (I'm still tired) I put more thought into what might have triggered this major FM event. I strongly suspect the chocolate but can't remember if I've eaten "hemp seeds" before.
6 days later	--	For breakfast I try ½ a muffin containing hemp seeds.
7 days later	--	I'm fine – it's was apparently the new chocolate that triggered my event. That brand goes onto my "avoid" list.

Now that I've laid the groundwork by defining the FM landscape let's look in greater detail at the specific triggering chemicals I've found and the compensations I use to manage them. Both topics have had major updates since I first wrote about them in 2011.

But first, let me lay my cards on the table in a way that will explain the rest of this book – what I've come to see as causing my FM pain and how I reached those conclusions.

Chapter Summary

- My fibromyalgia clearly stems from exposure to several modern chemicals.
- I call these "triggers' - not to be confused with FM trigger points.
- Other, "compounding factors" increase the degree and likelihood of pain but do not directly cause it.
- I'm able to compensate to a degree and avoid or diminish the pain.
- I'm calling the sequence from exposure through pain and recovery an "FM event".
- Pain and fatigue are my primary symptoms.
- An event begins with exposure (prolog) to the onset of pain (several hours later) through a gradual buildup and peak of pain (crescendo) and finally release, as the pain winds down.
- The pain can reach the level of a multi-day long migraine.
- Failure to control exposure leads to a continual level of pain that never lets up, a new "normal" - a certain base level of pain present at all times.

Why is this Happening?

With the increasing awareness I've developed over the past twelve years – especially after I sorted out most of the specific triggers that are associated with my FM events and began to control them – I have a firm, albeit lay, hypothesis as to what's going on. It's central to the sections that follow and lays the foundation for describing the factors behind all my years of pain.

There are multiple dimensions to Fibromyalgia as a condition that extends beyond the simple stimulus and response I see in my own body. These are the reasons I see behind its continued prevalence and why I don't expect relief to come any time soon – not simply the "what" but the "why":

Certain chemicals in food and the environment are, at least for me, "nerve irritants". Exposure to them – even in tiny amounts – results in the excitation of nerves that carry pain signals. The nerves in my head, face, nose, and mouth as well as my digestive system are stimulated in a way that results in irritation and, eventually, pain. Over time adjacent nerves become irritated as well as muscles and, eventually, results in the extreme pain of a full FM event.

It takes time for this to begin – hours after exposure – and it then builds from the initial irritation into a cascade effect that goes beyond the initial contact into a "pain for pain's sake" – some sort of sensitivity feedback storm – and takes hours to subside.

By avoiding exposure to certain physical substances, I can experience a complete absence of FM symptoms.

There are two exceptions to the need for a chemical trigger: the FM event that follows a bout with influenza or the cold virus and the event that follows a significant (prolonged) lack of sleep.

There are tentative signs of recognition in recent FM research that explores the effects of repeated bouts of pain and increased sensitivity but, at present, I'm left to my own devices. Avoidance of triggering chemicals is my best bet for avoiding FM.

I'm also concerned about additional dimensions to the Fibromyalgia condition that may explain the continued lack of treatment for chronic pain throughout the years I've been watching:

Pain simply isn't taken seriously, either in medical treatment or in research. I'm disappointed to continue to see disagreement over basic techniques of identifying and categorizing pain. We have a more robust system to categorize insect stings than for systemic chronic pain (see the Schmidt Sting Pain Index). The lack of an objective physical measure could be alleviated with social science techniques but is not. We need to view pain with the same spectrum-oriented approach used to describe the multidimensional aspects of alcohol abuse and its impact on our quality of life.

Death isn't the only bad health outcome we may experience – pain can be disabling and life-altering. Something broadly analogous to the Harm Reduction concepts of substance abuse combined with the economics of disability would better reflect the impact of chronic pain, rather than the "do or die" basis of so much current health research.

We're literally bathed in chemicals that were never robustly tested for their effects on life, human or otherwise. New compounds may be tested, but a long list of chemicals developed over the past two hundred years are simply accepted unless they have been identified as causing significant harm – largely defined as early death or serious physical disability. We're chipping away at these, the recent bans by the European Union on several food dyes is one example, but there's a long list that remains unexplored at this level of scrutiny.

To be fair, not all these substances are manufactured – several are natural spices, dyes, or flavorings, but the most impactful are human-engineered.

It's not always clear what substances we're being exposed to either in food or the environment. I strongly suspect that things make it into the food chain that are not reported in the standard list of ingredients seen on a product's packaging. I must be careful with any "new" food, even if it lists no ingredients I know as triggers. I strongly suspect they aren't always cumulatively identified – the raw materials used and listed have unlisted/unidentified components of their own that fail to make it to the formal ingredients list shown to the consumer. What consumers are aware of the cyanide compound in road salt?

It's difficult to get information on the various chemicals to which we are exposed. The global chemical tracking and reporting systems are well hidden from the consumer and, like the magical numbers reported on containers for "recycling" purposes, are largely defined by the entities who have an interest in maintaining the status quo. They'd like to continue to sell their products without interruption. The safety descriptions they write reflect their narrow self-interests.

Finally, and importantly, the fact that pain doesn't come quickly after exposure hides the relationship to a triggering chemical. The tendency of pain to be delayed 8 to 12 hours or more after exposure greatly complicates the identification of the factors behind pain. When you also consider that many simultaneously occurring triggers can be involved, that they are commonly occurring chemicals, and that it's difficult to clearly identify the ingredients in our food it's no surprise that we haven't identified these sooner.

I would also observe that **constant pain can become an accepted background state** – one that is only noticed when it spikes above the underlying lowest level. It took a brief pain-free period during summer vacation one year to awaken me to the fact that something was wrong and stimulate me to find a resolution. I had fallen into a trap where pain was simply a part of life, only the exceptional events were breaking through.

~

I've reached these conclusions after years of trial and error on my own body where each FM event was an experiment in the identification of a trigger. Accumulated success with pain reduction following my avoidance of suspected chemical triggers was a confirmation. Each failure leading to an FM event to which I could trace exposure to a suspect chemical was further proof that I was on the right track. Clarity only came with time and "natural experiment" after natural experiment.

No, I'm not able to define the physiological aspects underlying FM symptoms, but I know success when I see it on a daily basis. If I avoid these chemicals, I feel normal, if I fail to do so I experience FM events. Time and time again.

Triggers

To reiterate, I'm defining a trigger as something that directly causes my FM symptoms. Almost every pain event I experience can be traced back to a substance I ingest or I'm physically exposed to in some way.

Early on in my effort to understand and manage pain it occurred to me that a certain food dye - yellow 6, present in several baked products I favored, was somehow related to my discomfort. Fortunately, it had such strong effects I could readily see an improvement when I began to avoid it. I've described this period in detail in my earlier volume, "Coping with Fibromyalgia", suffice it to say it was eye-opening. Once I had realized that connection was possible, I continued to seek others, trying to think back at every FM event to ask what might have been the cause.

Several problems remained – I hadn't found all the possible triggers and I didn't have any way to manage the FM events that did occur. I wasn't convinced I had all the factors identified. The delay between contact and onset was confusing, making it hard to track back to any specific cause. The effects of an FM event interfered with the state of mind needed to analyze and identify potential new triggers. I still had a lot of disconnected ideas that I hadn't proven to my satisfaction.

My approach to finding these triggers has been simple: repeated trial and error. Once I recognized one substance as a trigger, I began to suspect there could be others. I continued to identify suspected influences, isolate them, and observe the results of avoiding them, over and over again.

Having experienced dozens of these events with this greater level of scrutiny it's now clear to me that exposure to certain substances will initiate an FM event. A chemical I ingest in food or that contacts my body initiates a response in me that I'm calling an "FM event". I simply don't experience the pain of FM events without an environmental trigger – exposure to a specific substance to which I'm apparently sensitive. I can now list those triggers with the authority gained from repeated experience.

Other factors may be involved in determining the degree of pain that results and how long it takes to recover – these include undue physical stress, poor posture, and eye strain – but there's no pain without an environmental trigger.

Triggers are cumulative – as in additive: exposure to two has a greater effect than one, and serial exposure to one has a greater effect than a single exposure.

Different triggers have somewhat different effects. Two, yellow 6 and nitrates, tend to quickly result in severe FM events. Others, such as road salt, take longer to show their effect. All are delayed somewhat, only showing an impact hours after exposure.

There are hints that these triggers are shared by others. They are beginning to turn up here and there in the FM reference materials as anecdotal references. Nitrates are mentioned, as is Earl Grey tea, at least as a trigger to the bare symptom of pain. The European Union is requesting several food dyes be avoided by food manufacturers – including yellow 6, though not as a trigger for pain. It has been banned for the past 20 years in Scandinavia.

While I readily admit I haven't performed basic research against a carefully selected sample of individuals, a heuristic approach has been highly effective for me. If I'm exposed to a trigger I experience pain, if not I experience pain-free normalcy.

~

I'll continue with a careful description of my triggers in the hope that they *are* shared – but read them with the understanding that your own may be different. We may not be sensitive to the same triggers. I doubt that I've found all the possible triggers that exist.

I'll start with a simple list of trigger factors and then expand on each one in turn. I've placed them in descending order of importance, or impact, as I perceive them. These can vary in their effects and in the techniques I use to avoid them, as well as in certain compensations I can take when I'm unavoidably or unexpectedly exposed to them.

Figure 1: Fibromyalgia Trigger Factors

- The food dye Yellow 6
- Chocolate
- Sodium Nitrate/Nitrite in cured meats
- Road salt
- Recovery from illness/lack of sleep
- Root Beer
- Earl Grey tea (bergamot orange)
- Additional suspected triggers:
    - Hair conditioner
    - Certain pesticides
    - Tire sealant (Slime)
    - Certain adhesives
    - Cloves and Annatto
    - Red wine
    - Soft drinks (Colas)

Chemical Trigger: Yellow 6

Description:

"Yellow 6" is a food additive that turns up in baked goods under numerous names, including Sunset Yellow FCF, FD&C Yellow 6, Orange Yellow, C.I. Food Yellow 3, Yellow Lake, and, in US food labeling, Yellow 6 or Yellow No. 6. In European food additive labeling it's denoted as E110. I'm using the "yellow 6" term because in U.S. food labeling that's how I often see it listed, if in fact it's shown at all.

I have known for years that this yellow dye is a strong trigger of my FM events – the strongest of them all when you consider the tiny amounts to which I'm exposed. It was the first factor I identified as "causing pain" – though at the time (the late 1970s) I had no more sophisticated understanding than that – I don't believe the term fibromyalgia had yet been coined. Avoiding it clearly helped reduce my episodes of "back pain" but didn't rid me of them entirely.

Finding a food ingredient that caused pain sent me on a decades-long quest to find other potential irritants – it was the first, and clearest source but not the only trigger. More were to come.

It's a synthetic dye made from coal tar and azo (a group of synthetic compounds characterized by vivid colors that are often used in dyes). It is currently banned in Norway and Finland and is among a list of six food colorings coming under increasing scrutiny in European Union countries where it has been linked to hyperactivity in children. The UK has asked for food manufacturers to voluntarily replace this and five other food dies with alternatives.

Its application has been in fermented foods that are heated (as in baked goods) as a control over color consistency. It's said to be used along with Amaranth (or with FD&C Red No. 3) to make a brown coloring that is sometimes used to control color consistency in chocolate and caramel – though I've never seen either of these listed in the ingredients of any chocolate product.

Yellow 6 is certified by the US Food & Drug Administration (FDA) as a food coloring additive to impart a yellow or orange hue to fermented or heated foods, including baked goods, candy, soft drinks, chips, and bread. In a typical 21st Century twist - it's also used to color common medications such as aspirin and antacids.

It has been tentatively linked to allergic reactions in people who have aspirin intolerance. The Washington D.C.-based Center for Science in the Public Interest called for the FDA to ban it citing research that identifies it as a potential carcinogen. The European Union requires products containing this dye to issue a warning that it could cause "an adverse effect on activity and attention in children".

I don't seem to have the same FM sensitivity to other, similar dyes such as FD&C Yellow No. 5 or Red 40, nor do I experience any of the commonly reported issues that people have with this food dye. Also known as tartrazine, Yellow No. 5 has been implicated in a variety of allergic responses, though this doesn't seem to include pain. I'm now suspicious of all food dyes and pay close attention to my exposure to them, but I can only claim to be sensitive to yellow 6.

The National Library of Medicine PubChem facility chemical safety category lists "Sunset Yellow FCF" (a.k.a Yellow 6) as:

Irritant

Note: PubChem lists 251 alias names for "Sunset Yellow FCF" including various forms of the terms FD&C, Yellow, and 6.

Effects:

I know of no concentration of yellow 6 that I can consume without triggering a significant FM event. Within a few hours of eating something that contains it I start to feel the onset of an event. It can be one of the strongest triggers, affecting my throat and neck first, which cascades into my shoulders and back as other muscle groups seem to be triggered to react.

I have no scientific basis for describing the adverse effects of yellow 6; I simply know that I need to avoid it like the plague. It's very clearly associated with triggering an FM event in me. Its clear and immediate effect was the likely reason it became the first FM factor I was able to identify.

Exposure:

Yellow 6 turns up in unexpected places, the product doesn't have to be noticeably yellow – it's apparently used to get the right shade of brown or tan. I've even seen it listed in the ingredients of a hot dog product.

Here it is listed in the "inactive ingredients" of a common aspirin product, apparently used in the yellow outer coating.

> **Inactive ingredients** corn starch, D&C
> yellow #10, FD&C yellow #6, hypromellose,
> methacrylic acid, microcrystalline cellulose,
> polydextrose, polyethylene glycol, shellac
> wax, silica, simethicone, sodium
> bicarbonate, sodium lauryl sulfate, talc,
> titanium dioxide, triacetin, triethyl citrate

And in a children's candy product (a red gummy treat):

> INGREDIENTS: SUGAR, INVERT SUGAR, CORN SYRUP, MODIFIED CORN STARCH, CONTAINS LESS THAN 2% OF TARTARIC ACID, CITRIC ACID, NATURAL AND ARTIFICIAL FLAVOR, YELLOW 6, RED 40, YELLOW 5, BLUE 1.

It's not always easy to find these – online retailers sometimes include a readable list of ingredients on their site pages, but many times they do not.

Compensations:

I must avoid this food additive at all costs, but avoiding it is a lot trickier than you might expect. I believe its inclusion in the source products that make up more complex foods is sometimes missed – as with my previous example of some chocolate products.

I'm a chocolate fan but must suspect any new source as being contaminated with Yellow 6. See the separate chapter that follows for additional detail on chocolate as a trigger.

Restaurant use is another source that's difficult to identify. I've come to suspect any unnaturally green, yellow, or orange ingredients as worthy of avoidance (orange dye can be a combination of red and yellow, green as yellow and blue). Salad dressings are a particular problem. As an example, I once ordered a salad with French dressing and, shortly thereafter, began experiencing the precursor symptoms. Its bright orange color should have alerted me to the possibility of trouble, and I remembered having the same reaction the previous time I ordered the same dressing in that restaurant. I also avoid Italian dressings based on similar experiences.

Food labeling laws and practices don't allow me to identify and avoid this trigger reliably. I simply suspect any yellow, green, or orange manufactured food items I'm not already sure about from trial and error. Its use in restaurants, especially in salad dressing, and as a hidden ingredient in some chocolate or cocoa is tricky to avoid.

Trigger: Chocolate

Description:

I'm listing "chocolate" as a trigger not because I suspect the basic ingredients– those created from cocoa beans - are a trigger for pain. Most of the chocolate products I've tried are perfectly safe for me. I'm instead listing it because certain chocolate products provoke a very strong FM reaction in me. I strongly suspect they contain the food dye yellow 6, added to improve or otherwise tailor the color of certain chocolate to the desired hue.

Until researching yellow 6 for this book I was unaware of its link to chocolate and caramel. I had harbored suspicions about chocolate for years but could never pin down the actual factor. I can tolerate chocolate (and cocoa) most of the time, but sometimes it seems that I can't. When I have problems with chocolate it feels the same as if I had been exposed to a strong trigger. Perhaps now I know why – I suspect that I can't handle it when yellow 6 has been used as a colorant in the basic ingredients.

It's also possible that the "Dutch process" for cocoa is involved with my sensitivity, where potassium carbonate, sodium carbonate, and/or sodium hydroxide may be used to alter the characteristics of this chocolate precursor. I've never seen these chemicals nor yellow 6 identified in the ingredient lists of chocolate products that have caused issues.

And finally, it's also possible that heavy metal contamination is to blame for my sensitivity, though in researching recent studies from Consumer Reports and others it's not a clear relationship. It's relatively rare for me to encounter "problem chocolate" while heavy metals seem to be found in many chocolates.

Effects:

This compound is one of the main sources of my major FM events – behind road salt. Chocolate is ubiquitous in food, and I've come to suspect dark chocolate as a trigger. Most dark chocolates are fine, some result in FM symptoms.

The effects I see with certain chocolates are identical to what I see when I'm exposed to the food dye yellow 6, a very strong FM event triggered by a very small amount of chocolate. See "the anatomy of a pain event" earlier in this book for an explicit description of just such an instance where I tried a chocolate product I had never before tasted.

Exposure:

Regardless of the underlying reasons, trying out a new source of chocolate is related to most of my unexpected FM events these days. I don't want to give up chocolate but never see yellow 6 listed in the ingredients so I'm tempted to try it to find out if I can tolerate it. I did so just before writing this paragraph and experienced a strong, 48-hour-long FM event.

Christmas is especially difficult given all the new chocolate sources with which I must contend. Yes, I could give up chocolate – but no, I don't want to give up chocolate. I'm careful to use known, safe brands and varieties – or pay the price in pain.

Compensations:

I've suspected chocolate and cocoa for some time in some FM events where I've ruled out other known triggers and a new chocolate product is in the mix, and yet I've never, not once, seen chocolate labeled with yellow dye as an ingredient. My suspicion is that it's present in some cocoa and/or chocolate sources – but its inclusion didn't pass through from the raw ingredient labeling (if there was any) to the final consumer product label.

The only realistic compensation I have for chocolate is to stick with previously proven safe products and to carefully test anything new.

Chemical Trigger: Sodium Nitrate/Nitrite

Description:

Many types of "cured" meat have the same effects on me as I see with yellow 6, provoking a strong FM event from even a minute exposure.

The kinds of cured meats that affect me include bacon, ham, hot dogs, luncheon meats, and the like. The common factor among them seems to be the food additives that are part of their manufacture. I strongly suspect the nitrates and/or nitrites used in that curing process.

I'm convinced it's the nitrate/nitrite additives because I *can* tolerate cured meats from organic sources that eschew the use of nitrates in their manufacturing processes. It was a tense meal when I first tried one of these – an organic ham - but it supported my hypothesis that nitrates are the trigger factor. I've experienced no FM symptoms at all after ingesting this specific brand of organic ham – one that advertised its lack of nitrates. I've moved on to other, similarly labeled cured and smoked meats – all without nitrates – without triggering an FM event.

Nitrates and nitrite compounds have historically been used in meat to control bacteria and impart a desired color and taste. They've come under increasing scrutiny as potential factors behind chronic pulmonary disease and in the formation of carcinogenic nitrosamine compounds when exposed to the acids of the stomach.

Wikipedia suggests that both sodium nitrite and sodium nitrate are used as curing agents in processed meats. They are available today from various sources as a food grade sodium nitrate or nitrite – often in a container that warns of hazards if contacted "directly" or used in other than recommended amounts.

I have had good luck in avoiding these chemicals as they are generally identified in the ingredients list of any food that uses them. Not all cured meats use them in their manufacture, but I've found it safer to assume that any cured meat includes nitrates and/or nitrites unless proven otherwise. The only caveat to this is found on web sites where cured meats are being advertised for sale. These often hide the ingredients, or at best make it difficult to find them. "Uncured" meats are often advertised with highly visible text, often in part of the description on the front of the package. Cured meats can be harder to identify.

At least four types of nitrate/nitrite compounds are used in food manufacture:

- Sodium nitrate
- Sodium nitrite
- Potassium nitrate
- Potassium nitrite

Other compounds are added to "food grade" sodium nitrite, including dyes to prevent confusing it with salt as well as "anti-caking agents" to preserve its pourability, but it's my experience that any cured meats containing nitrate or nitrite compounds provoke a reaction. I strongly suspect nitrates and nitrites rather than other additives.

I haven't performed an exhaustive study of which of these four additives trigger my FM pain – it's such as strong reaction I simply avoid all cured meats unless they advertise their lack of such additives, or I know they are free of them.

The National Library of Medicine PubChem facility chemical safety category lists both Sodium Nitrite and Potassium Nitrite as:

Oxidizer
Acute Toxic
Environmental Hazard

Sodium Nitrate and Potassium Nitrate are listed as:

Oxidizer
Irritant

Effects:

The impact and intensity of the FM-triggering effect of this food on me can perhaps best be illustrated by saying I can't even tolerate the bacon chips sprinkled on a salad. These are one of the most potent FM triggers I've ever experienced. It can simply knock me to the floor in pain within a few hours of exposure.

Cured meats were never a big part of my diet so it took longer to identify them as an issue.

Exposure:

Fortunately, nitrates generally turn up in expected places, various "cured" meats. I'm seeing increased availability of "uncured" products that specifically state, "no nitrates or nitrites added".

Here's an example from a "cured" ham product that includes both nitrates and nitrites:

Ingredients

Cured with Salt, Sugar, Brown Sugar, Sodium Nitrate, Sodium Nitrite

I've also seen nitrates/nitrites added to cured turkey products, canned "luncheon meats", and sadly, to SPAM.

Compensations:

At this point I simply stay away from any cured meat that I suspect of containing these chemicals. The few times that I've broken this rule have been catastrophic failures. I have a vivid memory of spending several hours at an interstate rest stop in great pain after indulging in a single-sliced ham sandwich at a conference luncheon where there were no alternatives on the menu. I was literally in too much pain to drive. I'm not highly motivated to experiment further.

Chemical Trigger: Road Salt

Description:

How can salt - applied to North American roads in huge quantities to foster safe and efficient driving conditions in the winter and eaten every day in every meal around the world – be related to my FM symptoms? Well, because road salt is not simply the chemical sodium chloride, that's why. It is salt that includes additives used to make it easier to handle – to prevent the natural caking process that would otherwise quickly turn the free-flowing salt grains into large salt blocks that would not flow freely through the road equipment used to apply it. These additives have included ferric ferrocyanide and sodium ferrocyanide. Ferric ferrocyanide is also known as Prussian blue – a dark blue pigment or dye, sodium ferrocyanide is often termed yellow prussiate of soda.

It's not easy to tease this information out of formal sources, it's well hidden. The entry for this compound in Wikipedia (as of this date, early 2023) no longer lists its use in road salt. It took a concerted effort to identify the components of road salt when I first became suspicious of that factor in 2004, it's even harder today in 2023.

A 2004 study for the Wisconsin Department of Transportation "Anti-caking Admixtures to Road Salt" (no longer available online) found only two additives in use in road salt based on a study of US States and these additives were the two ferrocyanide dyes listed above. It found evidence of hydrogen cyanide production under the combination of ferrocyanides, sunlight, and acid – (as in acidic rainfall). The current version of this document under the same name is far less specific - referencing the U.S. Environmental Protection Agency's designation of ferric ferrocyanide as a "toxic pollutant and hazardous substance" as well as concerns developing among Canadian researchers.

The blue variety – ferric ferrocyanide – isn't turning up in my area these days, thankfully, as it has a stronger and more immediate effect on me. If I'm correct in ascribing yellowish road salt to sodium ferrocyanide – then that's the variety that has been in use in my area (New England, USA) for the past ten years. That's corroborated by several (defunct and now unavailable) studies from U.S. state transportation departments as well as several local State Department of Transportation web sites where competitive bid data is made available.

At least one study has suggested that, under certain circumstances, these substances can break down in the environment and release free cyanide, a highly toxic chemical. Artist supply sites once suggested Prussian blue pigments "will emit toxic hydrogen cyanide gas if heated, exposed to ultraviolet radiation, or treated with acid" (though their current versions are much less helpful, issuing generic warnings in their Safety Data Sheet pages).

The effects of exposure to road salt aren't quite the same as for the prior two triggers I listed. Ultimately it has the same effect, an FM event, but the path there is somewhat more complicated.

Incidentally, the National Library of Medicine PubChem facility chemical safety category lists Sodium Ferrocyanide (a.k.a. Yellow Prussiate of Soda) as:

Acute Toxic
Irritant
Environmental Hazard

Effects:

I have a real and present issue with road salt. It is a clear and significant trigger factor that has caused many of my FM events. But to find this trigger it was necessary to reach a point where I was controlling all the other triggers.

It's not simply salt that I'm sensitive to. I live on the Atlantic coast and I'm regularly exposed to ocean salt and salt air, but I had never come to suspect it as an FM factor. I've been at sea for an entire day in exposed boats, at the beach, or on the rocks in heavy weather and exposed to salt spray repeatedly but never suspected that salt exposure was an FM factor. Yet, once I had many of the other factors under control, it was clear that road salt was a significant factor behind my FM pain.

Two scenarios are particularly bad: 1) during snowstorms when salt is applied and then turns to a wet, salty road surface and 2) after it has dried and becomes dusty. The dusty transfer of salt to my eyes, tear ducts and sinus cavity was understandable, but it took further research in aerosols to understand that salt can easily be transferred in the wet state to these same areas. That matched my experience exactly.

The effects of exposure to road salt are at their worst when it is first laid down but seem to decay somewhat over time. As the salt ages it seems to become somewhat less effective in triggering FM, though even relatively "old" spring salt can cause issues if I'm exposed to it long enough. This information isn't especially helpful because it's a challenge to know how old the salt is. It's laid down regularly throughout the environment as conditions change by multiple, independent public works units making it hard to assess its impact on me at any given time.

Salt applied during the deepest winter weather seems to have a somewhat less negative effect. I suspect that the colder conditions prevent the melting that leads to the kind of exposure that fosters my FM symptoms. These long-term cold spells are far less frequent these days in my area.

The worst exposure pattern (fastest onset of symptoms and strongest FM event) comes when salt is freshly laid down in melting conditions – as in early winter or late spring when snowstorms arrive but are immediately followed by fair weather and melting conditions. The wet, salty road conditions seem the best of all at causing symptoms. Traffic raises spray that, along with salt and its additives, is more readily transmitted to my eyes and nasal passages.

In the right conditions I even seem to be exposed inside my home and work environments. I must take care in sweeping out the garage as the dust seems to carry with it the previous season's road salt along with its irritant. One work location was near and below a busy street where, under the right conditions, road salt seemed to be carried into the office.

The long-term symptoms of exposure to treated road salt are like yellow 6 – but the earliest effects are different. Pain begins in my throat, face, and/or neck, migrating to my shoulders and back where the muscles seem to spasm in concert with the pain in my head. Symptoms begin to dissipate over time as the salt works its way out of my face. It's particularly impactful if I'm exposed for an extended period, as it seems to get into my tear ducts and takes longer to work its way out – providing a longer period of exposure. A long trip over dry, salty roads, a long walk at the roadside in breezy conditions, or a short exposure to freshly applied salt are all bad news.

Road salt exposure takes longer to result in FM symptoms than yellow 6. I may tolerate the first storm or storms but, after a few days of exposure and especially with repeated exposures over a series of days, the pain begins to appear. The effects are cumulative – daily exposure eventually leads to a point where my defensive measures can't keep up.

While it's hard for me to assess accurately I strongly suspect that I'm much more sensitive to ferric ferrocyanide (Prussian blue) than to sodium ferrocyanide. I once saw patterns of pain that changed over time, appearing to match the buying patterns of local public works departments rather than my own susceptibility. When I identified the presence of "blue salt" that I associate with ferric ferrocyanide I also noticed that I was affected more quickly and strongly with FM symptoms.

The recent EPA designation of ferric ferrocyanide as a toxic pollutant seems to have directed use toward the sodium ferrocyanide additive. Thankfully, I no longer see the characteristic "blue salt" being used on the highway (though it turns up occasionally on store walkways and stairs). Unfortunately, sodium ferrocyanide has the very same, if slower acting, effects.

Despite its less potent effects, road salt (sodium ferrocyanide) remains a leading cause of FM events – in part due to the difficulty of avoiding exposure.

Exposure:

Salt with sodium ferrocyanide turns up in many public places including local and state highways, parking lots and walkways.

When researching this chapter, I was unable to find a retail "rock salt" / de-ice solution using sodium chloride along with either of the ferrocyanide compounds. It's apparently limited to bulk sources used on public roads and/or parking lots – intended for use in our current mechanical spreading equipment. Retail melt products such as calcium chloride do not have the same adverse effects on me as "road salt".

Compensations:

Ideally, I will avoid exposure but since complete avoidance is not practical in this day and age, I'm often forced to "decontaminate".

Avoidance:

If I avoid exposure to road salt by staying off the highway when and where it's present in the environment, I'm unaffected by FM symptoms. If I venture outside again and become re-exposed symptoms recur. The absolute worst case for me is when I'm exposed for several hours, long enough for the salt (and presumably the cyanide compounds) to reach my tear ducts. I suspect by being transmitted to my eyes and wiped into the ducts the salt is then delivered slowly to my nose and throat where it becomes a long-term irritant. The resulting 12 to 24-hour period while the substances work their way out of my tear ducts and nasal passages can bring on a long-lasting FM event.

When I travelled to and from work daily (I'm now retired) I was re-exposed regularly – leading to regular bouts of pain. Now that I can control my exposure it's crystal clear that road salt causes FM events for me. It required this degree of control – the ability to stay home and avoid exposure – to finally prove to me that road salt was a trigger.

There's a season to road salt contamination that begins with its first application in the early winter and continues through spring. It takes significant rainfall to wash the salt off the roads – as in around six inches - so a relatively dry spring extends the pain season, a relatively wet one brings faster relief. Even weeks-old salt left behind after the previous winter use can cause pain if exposure lasts long enough (as in miles travelled on contaminated roads). One late freeze can start the process all over again as salt is reapplied to control icing.

Decontamination:

I simply treat road salt as if I were being exposed to radiation:

- I avoid road travel as much as possible or limit what I can't avoid.
- I wear a face mask while driving in salty conditions to reduce direct exposure.
- I "decontaminate" immediately after any exposure.

Here in northern New England, I'm forced to deal with exposure to sodium ferrocyanide for around six months of the year. I plan trips accordingly, wearing a mask while driving under salty conditions, doubling up on errands to reduce trips to a minimum, and giving myself time for "decontamination" after I return home.

My decontamination protocol includes the following steps:

- I wash my face as soon as possible after returning home.
- I use "natural tears" eyedrops to begin to rinse out my tear ducts.
- I use distilled water and a dedicated sinus rinse product to clear salt and sodium ferrocyanide from my sinus cavity (using nasal lavage).
- I take a shower to get the salt out of my hair and off my body as soon as I can.

If I begin these immediately after returning from a trip where I'm exposed, I can significantly reduce the resulting pain, if not avoid it entirely. Failure to follow the protocol predictably ends with an FM event, partially following the protocol triggers lower-level pain. There are no shortcuts to the steps above, for full relief it takes all the steps listed. Skipping steps means partial relief, at best.

When I was working, I saw noticeable (though not complete) success by taking the first two steps immediately after arriving in the morning and again after any further exposure during the day.

To perform nasal lavage, you rinse your nasal cavities with a mixture of distilled water and a salt/sodium bicarbonate solution. I'll list the one I use in the appendix. I've tried several but I found a dedicated kit with a premixed packet and applicator works best for me. I add distilled water and the contents of a pre-mixed packet to a specially designed bottle and rinse, following the enclosed directions.

Don't perform nasal lavage with tap water as it will act as an irritant and could introduce dangerous microbes into your nasal cavity, but with the proper solution it seems safe and is easily tolerated. This technique is not a perfect solution, but it clearly helps to reduce the effects of exposure to road salt's hazardous chemicals. It's ironic – rinsing with salt water to remove the road salt – but it can be effective at reducing FM symptoms caused by this trigger.

Road salt is not always as immediate a trigger as the others in the list of trigger factors, but it's so pervasive and unavoidable during the five months of winter here in northern New England –

December through March in most years - that it has a large overall effect.

Sadly, I have to say that road salt is the one factor I've had the least success in dodging. It's unavoidable during the winter months here in New England, under some conditions even invading my work and home environments. It often comes at the very time I'm under significant pressure from susceptibility factors such as high atmospheric pressure and relatively poor sleep (I seem to sleep best in spring/summer and fall, worst in winter). It has become the most impactful factor I'm unable to control and one that can lead to weeks of constant pain unless I take steps to control it.

Trigger: Recovery from Illness/Lack of Sleep

Description:

This is the single exception to the rule that I need to be exposed to an actual substance to trigger an FM event. After I've contracted a cold or influenza – as I begin to recover – I experience FM pain. This is quite predictable, coming before I've truly recovered from the original illness but near the end. Recovery from FM pain is coincident with recovery from the illness itself, coming as the symptoms from that incident subside.

I'm combining recovery from illness with lack of sleep as these two often occur together – I often sleep poorly when I have a cold or the flu. While this hasn't happened recently – I pay strict attention to getting proper rest - lack of sleep alone can eventually bring on an FM event. Fortunately, it takes several nights of poor sleep to result in FM symptoms. It's the rarest trigger I've listed here.

Effects:

This results in a "standard" FM event that's the same as any other from prolog through release.

Compensations:

Other than avoiding colds and flu there's not much I can do about illness as a trigger. The generic compensations I'll describe later are the best I can do.

Careful attention to "sleep protocol" was one of the first compensating actions I took – it had immediate and significant effects in reducing FM symptoms.

Managing coffee and caffeine is a related step I took, reducing the amounts I drank and keeping caffeine consumption to the mornings.

I also avoid decaf coffee – though not tea. There are several methods of removing the caffeine from coffee, but in my experience at least one of them clearly doesn't work for me. The last time I tried decaf coffee my sleep was disrupted for almost a week.

Chemical Trigger: Root Beer

Description:

This is the carbonated soft drink called Root Beer produced by numerous beverage companies across the world. It's not clear to me why I'm not tolerant of root beer, but it presents a problem and it's now something I avoid. It seems likely that one of its ingredients has an effect like those of the earlier trigger factors I've mentioned. Root beer flavoring has a rather lengthy list of ingredients with at least one, cloves, matching a known trigger.

As of this writing Wikipedia lists thirty-three potential ingredients in root beer added to induce foaming or as flavoring spices. If I were more of a root beer connoisseur, I might have greater motivation to identify the specific source and find a brand or source that eliminated it. As it is, I simply avoid it.

Effects:

This results in a "standard" FM event that's the same as any other from prolog through release.

Compensations:

I simply avoid Root Beer (and all other commercially prepared carbonated sodas, just for good measure).

Chemical Trigger: Earl Grey Tea

Description:

Earl Grey Tea? How can I pick on something as innocuous as this? Well, Earl Grey Tea, Lady Grey Tea, and some European candies contain a natural food constituent made from bergamot orange. Bergapten, a substance found in the oil of the bergamot orange, has been implicated as a potassium channel blocker – overconsumption has been identified as a source of muscle cramps (See the 2002 Lancet article "Earl Grey Tea Intoxication" *Finsterer J. Lancet 359:1484, 27 Apr 2002)*

All I can say with certainty is that I avoid products with bergamot because I've come to associate them with FM pain.

Effects:

Bergamot eventually results in a "standard" FM event that's the same as any other from prolog through release. It takes time, one cup doesn't seem to be enough to trigger pain, but it's clearly a trigger with cumulative effects that eventually lead to pain.

Compensations:

Again, regardless of the science behind bergamot, I find I'm much better off staying away from it. I might be able to tolerate a single cup – but I worry that it may add to my FM susceptibility. Over a period of days (and multiple cups) I have found it will reliably trigger FM symptoms. As with root beer I've simply given it up entirely.

Additional Suspected Triggers

I'm not certain about the impacts of these triggers but have strong suspicions about them. These also include substances where one component may be at fault, but I wasn't able to isolate it across two products. I'm simply not sure which of the many ingredients in these caused issues, so I'm avoiding or taking great care in handling them.

- Hair conditioner
- Certain pesticides (for example, ear mite medication for cats)
- Tire sealant (Slime)
- Certain adhesives
- Cloves and Annatto
- Red wine
- Soft drinks

I suspect each of these has triggered past FM events – so I avoid them.

I avoid **hair conditioner** after an especially painful episode. I purchased conditioner by mistake, rather than its associated shampoo in a similarly colored bottle and decided to try it. It took several sessions but became clear it was causing pain in my scalp. Discontinuing use discontinued the pain.

I'm suspicious of **pesticide** after a run-in with ear mite medication intended for my cat. Just a drop on my forearm was all that was needed to provoke pain. I've always been an organic gardener and so have little experience with these products.

I had a similar experience with a **tire sealant**, seeing pain on my forearm where some had settled.

At least one **adhesive** (a wood stove cement) triggered an event after it was applied and the stove heated for the first time.

I'm suspicious that I'm sensitive to **cloves and annatto** – at least in significant quantities. They turned up in certain energy bars I was eating, avoiding them helped. If cloves and annatto are involved, then they're less potent triggers than the rest. It took several meals to uncover these as potential irritants, but they're now on my avoidance list.

Cloves and annatto are turning up more frequently in energy bars, but here's a snapshot from the ingredient list from a vanilla ice cream.

IILK, PASTEURIZED CREAM, CANE SUGAR, I
(). ORGANIC ANNATTO EXTRACT (COLOR).

I've been suspicious of some **red wines**, but I rarely drink them and so lack the experience needed to tie this down. With red wine it seems possible that I'm feeling the effects of what is called "red wine headache" – sensitivity to something in certain red wines that results in headache symptoms. I don't encounter this often enough to avoid wine altogether, but it remains on my watch list. I rarely drink wine and seldom have issues when I do, so it's a difficult factor to track down.

It's been 15 years since I last drank commercially prepared **soft drinks** but at the time I gave them up I had strong suspicions that I was sensitive to one or more of their ingredients. It was clear that many root beer drinks caused issues, but I hadn't identified which specific ingredient in root beer or cola drinks might be causing issues. There are plenty to choose from including flavorings, preservatives, colorings, or artificial sweeteners. These suspicions were not the only reason I gave up commercial soft drinks – I was also concerned by the amount of sugar they contain and the untested, risky nature of artificial sweeteners. I felt that I didn't need the huge number of nutrient-free calories they added to my diet. It was simply easier to give them up and find something else to drink than to sort out all the ingredients and accept the risks of artificial sweeteners.

~

I'm less certain of these triggers in this "other" category because I've been able to avoid them. As with other foods that I've come to suspect as FM factors, I'm not highly motivated to engage in extensive testing of my own to identify the specific ingredient that is at fault. It's easiest to simply give up a suspect food entirely.

If I *were* motivated then it would take a long series of careful tests controlling which sodas I drank, watching to see if any symptoms followed, giving them up entirely for some time, and watching for improvements in symptoms – all the while taking care to note my exposure to any known FM factors that could skew the results. I would also look for those brands that had the fewest additives, perhaps looking for an "organic" or local source.

Rather than doing that work I now make my soda from pure carbonated water. I originally used store-bought seltzer, now I even create my own carbonated water from tap water and bottled carbon dioxide gas in a home-carbonation machine. I control the ingredients, finding I don't need to add any sugar and can use simple, raw flavors without preservatives, colorings, artificial sweeteners, or whatever else modern marketing might suggest.

Chapter Summary

- Common triggers of pain include:
    - Yellow 6 (under numerous names) a widely used food dye used to turn food yellow/brown/orange/green.
    - Chocolate – possibly when it's dyed with yellow 6.
    - Sodium nitrate/sodium nitrite a widely used meat preservative in hot dogs, ham, bacon, and luncheon meats.
    - Sodium ferrocyanide – an additive used to condition "road salt" for use in salt spreading equipment.
    - Recovery from illness/lack of sleep. Both can trigger an FM event.
    - Root beer, Earl Grey tea (bergamot), cloves, annatto, and others.
- Avoidance is the ideal compensation - "decontamination" is required for road salt as avoidance isn't always practical.

Compounding Factors:

Compounding factors are those things that can make an FM event more severe, but which generally do not result in an event without an actual trigger being experienced. I'm calling these compounding factors as they seem to increase the amount of pain I'm experiencing, as well as increasing the likelihood of reaching a full-blown FM event.

I termed this "susceptibility" in my earlier book, to describe my general predisposition to experience an FM event. How likely am I to experience pain on any given day? At that time, I suspected these compounding factors could trigger an FM event without exposure to a trigger factor. I needed to find and confirm the last trigger before it became clear these merely contribute to the severity of the pain – a trigger was needed to set things in motion.

It took time for me to sort out the triggers from compounding factors – with road salt as the major complication. The effects of road salt are less immediate and weaker than the other major factors (yellow 6 and nitrates) and so were harder to pin down in the earlier stages. It was also exceedingly difficult to control – it took the enforced isolation of the Covid-19 era and the privileges of retirement to result in a proper natural experiment that allowed me to completely avoid this trigger – and to clearly identify it as a trigger.

If you read the first volume "Coping with Fibromyalgia" you'll see that I didn't understand the ongoing, underlying effects of road salt, resulting in a more complicated view of the steps needed to manage FM pain. I saw it as a balance to be maintained between a broad and intricate set of compensating actions and pain triggers, with susceptibility as an ongoing mediator. It's now clear to me that I need one of the triggers listed earlier to fall into a FM pain.

I was also missing the varying levels of pain that I can experience. Not all FM events are alike – they don't all take the classic form and progress to extreme pain. Some simply result in ongoing discomfort of varying degrees. That's especially true now that I have triggers under control – I can now compensate in several ways to avoid or minimize exposure. It's only the rare event today that breaks through unexpectedly and leads to a full-blown FM event.

Triggers and these compounding factors are cumulative – greater exposure can add up to increased pain and/or a full FM event. I've learned to keep a running tally in my mind, just what compounding factors are in effect at any given point in time and at what scale? Triggers, on the other hand, are to be avoided at all costs, in any amount. They needn't be accompanied by compounding factors; they always bring FM symptoms when they are experienced.

And yet susceptibility remains a valid description of my underlying resistance to pain. FM events that occur from exposure to a trigger factor are more severe when I'm under the influence of multiple compounding factors. I continue to manage these factors as part of my active coping strategy even though they take a back seat to avoidance.

Figure 2: Compounding Factors

- High atmospheric pressure
- Mental stress
- Cold weather
- Lack of restful sleep
- Daylight saving time
- Undue physical stress
- Poor posture

High Atmospheric Pressure

Fast changing low to high atmospheric pressure often brings on the increasing tension I've come to know as the precursor to FM. Either an extended period of high pressure or a fast change to a higher or lower state can influence my susceptibility.

The combination of this factor with exposure to road salt can be a problem, such as when an early spring storm passes through with a cold front just behind it. The road salt is bad enough – but the increased susceptibility that the rapid change to high pressure brings can make things even worse.

There's not much I can do about this factor except to be aware of its presence at any given point in time. It tilts the balance toward FM and means I must take it easy and start thinking about how to begin compensating. I can then pay more attention to the factors I *can* control.

Mental Stress

Certain kinds of psychological and emotional stress can contribute to my FM susceptibility. These are generally not the normal stresses of life, but those I would call unusual.

I'm including a variety of mental stresses in this category – in part because I'm not qualified to identify them in medical terms. Suffice it to say stress at work or home can contribute to my susceptibility like the other factors in this overall category.

Overwork, uncertainty at work, a death in the family, conflict, or other similar events increase the severity of symptoms. Certainly, this is true if the stress is severe enough to interfere with sleep and bring in that factor, but it can also have negative effects at lower levels of impact.

It's not just extraordinary or unusual pressures I'm talking about here, it's also the sum of everyday stresses at work and home that we all feel in this fast-paced, in-your-face, and connected world. As an example – I gave up watching (or listening) to the news regularly. I still read the newspaper but pay attention to the effects of even that exposure to the world.

It was Dr. Andrew Weil who suggested in one of his health columns that you will hear about anything really important, you don't need to stay connected to every single news item daily. He was right – I'm not missing anything by skipping the nightly news, I hear about the truly important things and can follow up on them when I feel the need. The constant attention to "bad" news – at least in my case – contributed to my overall level of stress. I continue to get my news from written sources where I have greater control over my exposure, but strictly limit what news I follow in the electronic media.

It's not only the news that induces an underlying stress in me – much of what passes for entertainment on television has, at its heart, the goal of catching and holding our attention. It does so by over-emphasizing all aspects of its message: all news is bad news, every event is the event to end all events, every celebrity misstep is the end of entertainment as we know it, and so on.

And it doesn't end there – the very tone and flow of every moment of modern television and film is tailor-made to catch and hold attention, never letting up on the volume, intensity, or rhythm – carrying us into and through the real goal of the medium: exposure of our attention to the subtle messages of the advertisers.

I'm not a sports or talking head fan, but I can see the same patterns played out in this content, as well. Their constant forceful and focused sound and image have their intended effect on me - catching and holding my attention.

I'm convinced that the modern media, especially "anger entertainment", are a compounding factor all on their own. I include them here under "mental stress" because I believe that's the effect they have on me (one I see reflected in others). I need to manage my exposure to this media a contribution to the negative side of the FM balance sheet. As such I pay attention to what I'm being exposed to and avoid the worst offenders of the calm.

I find myself asking "what am I getting from this?" when watching any of the modern media sources. If the answer is "not much" then I move on.

The media is not the only cause of stress in my life, of course. All the traditional causes stemming from emotional uncertainty and conflict as well as the physical stress of overwork are also to blame. All of these contribute to my susceptibility to FM and need to be managed as part of the ongoing balance I need to maintain in order to remain well.

Cold Weather

Cold weather in and of itself appears to be a factor behind my FM sensitivity. It's compounded by the presence of other factors such as road salt, short daylight hours, and strong weather patterns that accompany cold weather in the northeast, but it remains a time of greater susceptibility for me. Now that I've found many of my trigger factors the spring, summer, and fall months are much less painful, but winter remains a trying time - particularly during the coldest few weeks in December through early February.

Dressing warmly doesn't seem to help with this factor; it seems to be a result of my body's response to the changes in climate that cold weather brings, rather than a one-for-one relationship between becoming cold and experiencing symptoms, although cold alone can be a problem, as in sitting too close to an air conditioning source. Generally, the kind of FM pressure that a draft would bring is an aggravation rather than the significant complicating factor that cold weather represents.

It may also be the perfect storm of factors that seem to occur in winter that lies at the root of this: including the increased prevalence of strong high-pressure systems, their faster onset in winter months, exposure to road salt, and a decrease in restful sleep that the winter months always seem to bring.

I may be reacting to seasonality here – my sensitivity to the day-length changes and lack of sunlight we experience in the higher latitudes of northern New England. While I don't experience the complete set of symptoms described as

Seasonal Affective Disorder (SAD) I can relate to its timing and sleep disruption aspects.

My own FM season – the months when I experience the greatest pain – did once tend to match the calendar quite well. The November through March period was the height of pain for me for many years. These are the months when exposure to road salt is possible, depending on specific weather conditions. It's also the time of year when I face the greatest challenge of getting restful sleep, as well as a time when my traditional compensations work less well. The actions that would normally prevent FM symptoms in another season fail to have as strong an effect in the winter months. I experience most of my FM events in winter.

On the other hand, warm weather (and warmth itself) seems to help reduce my susceptibility and symptoms. I feel much better throughout the few warm months we have here in the northeast, and even more so during hot spells in the depth of summer (a few weeks in July and August here in New England).

I can't remember a truly hot summer day when I've had an FM event, at least in recent years when I've gotten so many trigger factors under control. Trigger factors can break through even that defense so hot weather is not a panacea, but in general hot weather brings an added degree of relief from or resistance to what would otherwise result in a problem.

I'm also able to use warmth as a compensation technique, as in heated seats in a vehicle or a hot shower. I'll describe its use in greater detail in the next chapter.

Lack of Restful Sleep

Lack of sleep might be a trigger in and of itself if I didn't pay such strict attention to it. It was the factor first tackled by my physician and one that continue to take very seriously. It's a chicken and egg scenario – pain can interrupt sleep; lack of sleep clearly compounds the pain of any FM event. Establishing an effective "sleep protocol" was a core part of my early FM remediation efforts and is covered in greater detail in the Compensations chapter.

Daylight Saving Time

I find both the fall and spring time changes to move on and off "daylight saving time" to be stressful, interrupting my sleep pattern and adding a stress factor that contributes to my FM susceptibility.

Now that I'm retired, I'm in a much better position to react to these changes, altering my sleep patterns a week before the switch in an attempt to slip into the new routine. Despite these measures the time changes remain a stressful experience.

Undue Physical Stress

By "undue physical stress" I mean exercise or physical activity that causes significant muscle soreness. It can also mean inattention to posture that leads to strained or overused muscles. The soreness and pain that reaches my back, shoulders, and/or neck is particularly bad when it affects the same muscles that are involved in an FM event, compounding its effects.

Poor Posture

Posture is related to the pain I might experience in an FM event. It's easy to overlook this, but it's significant for me as a modern office worker having sat at a computer terminal for over 40 years using a keyboard and mouse. Many of the muscles involved in my FM events are the very same ones taxed by the demands of the keyboard and mouse.

While it's often associated with occupational health and safety, posture is just as important a factor when you are away from work. As an example, long driving sessions can be a problem for me, especially in an unfamiliar or uncomfortable vehicle or at a time when other susceptibility factors are at play. Driving also requires using the same muscles that are involved in an FM event and so risks stressing these and triggering FM. (It also exposes me to road salt when that factor is in season.)

Paying attention to ergonomics has paid off for me – both in an occupational sense (the layout and physical setup of my space at home and work) and in a more general sense, including the same layout issues at my home computer and in all the other places I spend time, such as chairs, my home workbench area, and automobiles. I'm writing this at a standing workstation, one that can be raised or lowered at will – but once I began using it, I've never lowered it. I prefer standing, even for extended periods (though that can take some getting used to).

Posture is also a factor in everyday life when reading, eating, watching television, or seated in a restaurant. Those are the times I need to pay the strictest attention to my body position, especially if I am under the influence of an FM factor and beginning to feel the precursor symptoms of an FM event.

There are several posture-improving programs available to deal with this in an organized fashion. I won't repeat these here, but instead refer you to several articles by Jane Brody in the New York Times – please see the Resources section for a link.

Chapter Summary

- "Compounding factors" can make FM events more likely or severe, but don't trigger events all on their own.
- These factors include:
    - high atmospheric pressure
    - mental stress
    - cold weather
    - lack of sleep
    - daylight saving time (the changes)
    - physical stress
    - poor posture

Compensations

*[This chapter is largely unchanged from the "Coping with Fibromyalgia" book with **one major exception: the use of TENS** (Transcutaneous electrical nerve stimulation) once pain begins].*

In my earlier book "Coping with Fibromyalgia" I wrote a long "Compensations" chapter, with an extensive list of actions I found helpful in avoiding, deferring, and/or reducing the effects of FM. I was coming from a state of nearly constant pain, managing it to acceptable (lower) levels was the best I could do at the time.

Finding all the sources of my FM pain has turned things around completely. Rather than constantly planning for its inevitability I'm now able to go for long periods pain-free. Pain is now the exception rather than the rule.

Everything I wrote in that earlier "Compensations" chapter remains true and useful, and I'd recommend reading it for its historical and situational value – it describes a certain state I had reached, one you may be in today.

In the Triggers chapter I described the specific actions I take to avoid and/or react to each of the chemicals I know trigger my FM symptoms – but there are other, more generic actions that I take that I haven't covered yet in any detail.

These are the things I do to prevent, delay, or recover from an FM event or to reduce its severity and length – that is, to correct or adjust for its impact on my life. It's a rather broad set of behaviors, techniques, and actions and includes an ongoing effort to better understand the factors I've mentioned in the previous chapter and to identify any new ones I may have overlooked. I'll describe this research aspect in a later chapter, focusing here on the behaviors, techniques, and actions I have already found.

In this chapter I'm closer to traditional FM literature, but I still find it necessary to provide my own terms and definitions. While many of the things I do to mitigate the pain of FM come directly from existing FM sources I see compensation in broader terms. By "compensate" I mean taking actions to avoid, reduce, or correct FM pain. It's a different list than I've seen in other sources, including but not limited to the traditional FM pain relief measures. It also includes some unusual ways of dealing with an FM event, techniques I've found helpful and haven't seen documented elsewhere.

You'll note that I don't describe any of these compensations as cures – because they don't prevent all my FM symptoms. They do reduce them greatly, to such an extent I feel I live a very normal life, colored as it is by the need to adjust at times for what would otherwise result in an FM event – to change my behavior in various ways that I've found can reduce the incidence and severity of FM symptoms.

In general, these compensations are characterized by the need to pay close attention to my ongoing physical state, avoid the triggers I've come to know result in FM symptoms, and by the need to react quickly to the precursor symptoms I've come to associate with a developing FM event.

I've had no success with over-the-counter pain relief products and had particularly poor results with pain relievers that include caffeine or other stimulants. I believe this was because they disrupted my sleep. My FM pattern - where I mainly have pain in the evening - meant that to use them effectively I was ingesting caffeine precisely at the very moment it was least appropriate, interfering with the restful sleep I need to maintain my balance and thus perpetuating the very cycle I was trying to break.

I didn't find this out without trying a lot of OTC non-prescription pain relievers – I'll omit the list here, but the widely advertised OTC pain relievers were the first thing I tried many years ago and repeated unsuccessfully many times since then. Most of these attempts, I'm convinced, resulted only in making things worse. I can't provide a clinical explanation of why this is so for me – but I don't need to. Repeated experiments where I've tried and failed have shown me that they offer me very little relief. Your experience may differ, but I rarely use OTC pain medications. When I do it's not for dealing with FM symptoms, it's for more traditional pain such as that of a pulled muscle.

To be clear – some of these OTC pain relievers, especially those with caffeine, *can* reduce pain for a time. Unfortunately, their overall effect on me is negative when they disrupt my sleep and bring on a second round of FM pain even more severe than the first. This leads to a downward spiral from which it is not easy to break free.

It is also necessary to pay attention to the inactive ingredients of these pain medications because they can include some of the very dyes and additives that I've come to suspect as FM factors. I've found that house brand pain relievers with the same active ingredients as the name brands often come with a lighter load of marketing components such as dyes. They also come in a purer form, containing only the active ingredient intended for pain relief without the extra components such as caffeine.

All this is not to say I have no pain relievers in my home because I do, but I only seem to need them if I pull a muscle or do something similar that results in "normal" pain. The traditional uses for OTC pain relievers work for me, but they fail to relieve my FM symptoms. I haven't given up trying to treat FM pain using the new OTC pain relievers coming on the market. Provided I can find them in a relatively pure form I'll try them on occasion. I've yet to find something I feel works regularly, but I also know how complicated this can be. It can take repeated trials to be sure something truly doesn't work, including trials in varying circumstances of pain, across different brands, and in different doses.

At this point I've had so little success with OTC pain relievers I'm leaving this category off the list of compensations entirely. I can't say anything definitive about how they impact my FM symptoms except to point out where they have failed – by including ingredients that indirectly complicate matters for me (caffeine and other stimulants) or that introduce risk by including inactive ingredients that I've come to suspect as potential FM factors in and of themselves.

As for prescription pain relievers I'll only say that I'm deeply suspicious of any substance that could result in my becoming addicted to it. While I can completely understand the compelling business justifications of a product that predictably retains its customer base, I fail to see the benefit of simply trading one monkey on my back for another - not to mention the potential physiological side effects of these drugs. No, I'll pass on these until I see a safer return for my investment – so to speak.

The compensations that work best for me are a rather eclectic list of behaviors and activities that don't seem to share anything much in common – except that engaging in them has, for me, the effect of reducing or even heading off the progression of FM pain. Some of these come right from the FM literature, but some I've stumbled onto by accident.

To better describe these compensations I'm going to separate them into two categories: those actions that should be started before FM symptoms begin to appear (and continued after they appear - that is, before any of the precursor symptoms are present and when managing an approaching or active event), and actions to be taken after symptoms begin to appear. The measures to be taken during these two phases of FM are quite different. The former are measures that are intended to head off the pain and the latter are measures to deal with its presence. Both sets of actions are required – neither, alone, is enough to manage my FM symptoms.

In practice, I tend to work with all these measures reflexively, in a kind of ongoing management effort that deals with whatever the risks are at the moment and become more active at the first sense of an oncoming FM event. There's an element of balance involved, trading off compensations against factors I've been exposed to recently in the demands of daily life. It has become a part of who I am and how I respond to the world around me.

For the sake of description, I'll organize these into the categories shown in figure 3.

Figure 3: Compensations

Before symptoms appear:

- Getting restful sleep
- Avoiding trigger factors
- Maintaining FM situational awareness
- Managing stress
- Exercise and posture

After symptoms appear:

- Managing an oncoming FM event
- Using TENS - Transcutaneous electrical nerve stimulation
- Coping with the pain of an active FM event
- Recovering from an FM event

Compensations before FM symptoms appear:

These compensations are in keeping with my goal of heading off FM events before they occur. If I'm proactive with the knowledge I've gained over the years I can use it to head off symptoms before they appear.

Getting restful sleep

Sleep is the single most important compensation I must work with against the pain of fibromyalgia and one of the earliest factors I identified. It's a complex factor for me because it has two contrasting aspects: experiencing restful sleep contributes significantly to my resistance to all the other factors that promote FM symptoms, but failing to get adequate and proper sleep may become a trigger factor on its own.

Sleep is both a factor that must be managed to avoid its contribution to FM and a compensation that can be applied to reduce the probability of any other factor becoming an influence. Failing to get restful sleep can eventually result in minor FM-like symptoms. Getting proper restful sleep can provide resistance to some of the weaker-acting FM factors.

Getting the correct kind of restful sleep regularly boosts my ability to resist FM - at least from factors that I might expect to result in minor symptoms, such as an approaching high-pressure system. It's not a cure-all, trigger factors can still break through even if I'm otherwise getting restful sleep on a regular basis, but it provides resistance to the less impactful factors.

I first became aware of sleep as a factor when it was suggested by my physician. It was during my initial visit where I presented the information I had gathered on the internet about fibromyalgia and said to him "this looks a lot like me". He had stepped away for a few minutes to read and absorb the material I brought and then returned to ask a single, pointed question: "do you get restful sleep?" It sounded like an easy question to answer, but I hesitated and was led to ask myself the question more seriously. I had to admit that I couldn't answer with a clear "yes – I do get restful sleep".

The answer quickly developed into a clear "no" when I began taking medication to address the issue. The very first morning after taking the medication I awoke to realize that I had not been sleeping well at all. I had forgotten what it was like to sleep soundly – I awoke on that first morning feeling truly refreshed in a way that was new to me. After only a few days of truly restful sleep I realized that my FM symptoms were beginning to improve dramatically.

I had fallen into this state slowly enough not to have noticed it. There was no single point in time when I suddenly began sleeping poorly. Over time a lack of restful sleep had slowly become normal.

When I was able to begin managing this factor by getting truly restful sleep it began my journey out of pain and into the world of relative normalcy. As soon as I began to sleep soundly, I began to see a reduction of FM symptoms and the recovery process began that I described in an earlier chapter. It's not the whole story. Restful sleep doesn't protect me from FM pain and getting restful sleep requires a constant and determined effort.

I also began to pay a lot more attention to basic sleep protocol – taking steps to avoid the kinds of activities that seem to interfere with restful sleep, getting exercise, and generally following the advice of several sleep clinics and support groups. Paying greater attention to sleep meant developing an approach – a sleep protocol – that I use regularly.

I went into this in greater detail in "Coping with Fibromyalgia", describing a rather long period beginning with a sleep enhancing medication

(Amitriptyline), and gradually reducing that until it was no longer needed, all the while ramping up basic sleep measures and exercise, managing caffeine and diet until I reached a point where sleep was working out well for me.

The key to your sleep may be different, but for me it includes:

- Going to bed and waking at the same time each day (within an hour or so).
- Avoiding stimulating television or radio for a few hours (at least an hour) before sleeping. This is a challenge – all television is intended to be stimulating these days in a vast grab at our attention, to prevent us from changing channels, to keep us glued to the set between shows and to coax us to pay attention to the commercial content in advertisements.
- Not reading, eating, or watching TV in bed. Using the bedroom for sleeping.
- Eating carefully. I'm kept awake if I eat too much at dinner (the last meal of the day) or eat a meal that is too high in carbohydrates. I wake up during the night if I have too much sugar or another strong carbohydrate in the afternoon or evening. (I follow the Zone diet closely and when I do so I can avoid these issues).
- Fasting overnight – with no snacking after my last meal around 6 PM.

- Drinking carefully. Alcohol is a strong carbohydrate and can have the same effect on me as sugar – so I drink no alcohol at all. Drinking too much liquid interferes with an uninterrupted night's rest by forcing me to awaken and empty a full bladder. Drinking caffeine late in the day interferes with my sleep.
- Controlling light sources, even including my clock radio, to maintain near darkness.
- Wearing earplugs to reduce the impact of sounds throughout the night.

One other sleep-related technique that I find helpful is to sleep with a "shallow" pillow. I have tried a lot of pillows over the years, but a few years ago I settled on using a very thin one, and it seemed to make a significant difference. It took some getting used to – it results in different sleep positions than I would otherwise adopt when using a normal pillow - but it results in a major improvement in my sleep.

Working through sleep issues was one of my earliest and most impactful compensations. I continue to pay attention to sleep as, at its worst, it can trigger FM symptoms all on its own.

Avoiding trigger factors

The second most significant compensation I've found to prevent the occurrence of FM symptoms after restful sleep would be to simply avoid exposure to those factors that I've come to know cause or "trigger" them in me.

Admittedly all this is really saying is "if it hurts when you do that, don't do that" but it's not an easy task to avoid the trigger factors I've come to know as the cause of my FM events. I might easily forget that I'm sensitive to a component in root beer and have some. I'd remember soon enough, as it has a relatively fast onset of effects – but it's easy enough to forget over a period of years that something is a trigger factor. I simply try to maintain awareness of the list of trigger factors I've come to know.

The actions I take to avoid and compensate for triggers are specific to each individual one and so are explained in the trigger chapter, above.

Maintaining FM situational awareness

Another way I maintain my FM balance is by maintaining an awareness of my physical state and the factors that influence it. It's a kind of FM-specific situational awareness, – more than simply being aware of my current level of pain, my susceptibility, and the factors I've been exposed to recently.

Finding that chemical triggers are the root of nearly all my FM pain has focused my attention on the "exposure" side of the equation. That requires a certain constant awareness of what I'm eating and doing with a retroactive perspective, something we don't normally do. Who remembers what they ate at each meal the previous day? Yet it was critical to finding the chemical triggers I now know affect me adversely.

Every pain episode requires this retroactive review of what I've been up to recently. If that wasn't complicated enough – I need to separate out "normal" pain from "FM pain". I've become much better at it, FM pain has unique characteristics, but there's some overlap between the two sources.

So - I pay more attention to each meal and try to anticipate problems. I have a running list of potential triggers that I apply to any new food. I go for long periods eating only those things I've come to know and trust (though changes in their ingredients can and have tripped me up). I'm also forced to look with care at new foods – something especially difficult during all the holidays. My aunt's prize roast ham is out of bounds – finding a way to skip it is no easy task. July 4th hot dogs – verboten and no easier to pass up.

In short, I can't afford to forget that I'm afflicted with fibromyalgia and need to take measures most everyone else can ignore. Implementing them can be a sociological conundrum with no easy answers.

Managing stress

I've come to see stress as an important contributor to the level of pain I would otherwise experience with FM. I covered this in detail in my earlier book and so I'll just summarize here. It's also a well-known contributor so I have little to add to what's already published on the subject.

Suffice it to say – I pay attention to stress as an FM factor. It had much more relevance when I was working, but I continue to think of stress reduction as a compensation I need to make.

Exercise and posture

The link between exercise and the reduction of FM symptoms was apparently one of the first compensations uncovered by medical researchers when the condition was becoming accepted. Several early authors suggested it might be possible to overcome symptoms completely if only you could get enough exercise.

In my own experience exercise clearly reduces my susceptibility to FM. It was my earliest compensation – the first thing I tried after finding the yellow dye/pain link and beginning to take FM seriously as something I needed to deal with. I began with walking on a treadmill, gradually expanding over the years into a more varied routine.

Aside from feeling better in general, if I maintain an active routine by getting at least three exercise periods each week my symptoms are reduced in frequency and severity.

There are many fine exercise plans out there – I use the plans and guidelines published by the American Heart Association – I'm sure there are many more that can lead to fitness while taking other health factors and conditions into effect.

What works best for me is to vary my exercise sources constantly so that I don't become too bored with the same activities performed repeatedly. As an example, I have a rowboat and enjoy rowing, I mow the lawn with a hand mower, shovel snow by hand (for the first 20 – 30 minutes, at least), walk, and hike. I have a general goal of 20 to 30 minutes every other day, never going more than two days without an exercise period that brings my heart rate up to at least the point where I would find it hard to talk normally.

Posture requires similar dedication to maintaining awareness of how my body position over time results in an overall state of tension or relaxation. It demands its own balance sheet but requires more immediate changes when I sense things beginning to tense up. It requires greater attention if the overall balance is tipped toward FM and I'm beginning to experience its early symptoms.

I'm defining posture broadly - as the position of my body in space and in the stresses and strains maintaining that position can bring. It's not limited to industrial ergonomics – it's more than simply paying attention to my seated position – it's the way I carry and hold my body's position at all times, when seated and working or reading, when standing, when walking, when driving a vehicle, when riding in a vehicle, when fishing, when sleeping or napping.

The common theme between all these positions is the stress that can arise from holding my body in the same place for a long period. To me the impact of this stress seems much like FM itself, rather difficult to define precisely, but a kind of discomfort that starts with a more innocent uncomfortable feeling that, unheeded, develops into greater discomfort and a more traditional kind of pain. Pain that can add to the more classic symptoms of a full FM event. It's important to pay strict attention to the effects of posture throughout the day (and night, with your sleeping position). If something hurts, make changes early and often. Pain is not normal; if it's present then something needs to be moved, stretched, relaxed or adjusted.

Helpful information on posture seems somewhat hard to find. I've cited a Mayo Clinic link in the Resources chapter and further information is available by searching the terms "back pain" on this site and others, but I've never found a comprehensive treatment of "posture" that satisfies my needs. The discipline of ergonomics covers seated posture and common work challenges well but leaves out the day-to-day aspects of posture I find most challenging. I've included two Jane Brody articles from "The New York Times" in the Resources section that include additional information on the importance of posture.

In addition to the specific recommendations on posture offered here I would add two more things: regular stretching and specific body trunk exercises. Both are needed on a regular basis (weekly, at the very least). I find that stretching is particularly important in the winter months.

By "body trunk exercises" I mean specific strength training in the muscles in my neck, shoulders, back, and waist. These exercises include sit-ups, pushups, and a kind of reverse sit-up that strengthens my lower back and contributes to better posture. This is performed by lying face-down on the floor and raising both head and feet from the floor at the same time.

The combination of stretching and exercises reduces back pain in general, whether directly related to FM symptoms or not.

"Sleeping posture" is another important measure to consider. The term may sound odd, but the positions I assume during sleep are related to pain – both as a remedy and as a cause. There are numerous sources available that describe how to approach the sleep position, let me just say that I take it very seriously. I pay attention to my sleeping position and change it when I'm not completely comfortable. I pay particular attention to becoming comfortable when I first go to bed as it seems like this comfort carries through overnight. This may be another case of discomfort creeping into my life slowly – and unnoticed. Uncomfortable sleep can slowly become the norm without our becoming aware of it.

Exercise and posture are closely related and are significant factors behind my FM pain. Both can contribute to or reduce my susceptibility to FM pain and need to be managed carefully.

Compensations after FM symptoms appear:

These are compensating actions I take after FM symptoms begin to appear.   It's a very different list than the more generic steps I had been taking all along, and generally begins with the onset stage when I realize it's FM pain that's occurring rather than some more straightforward source.

Managing an approaching FM event

At his point I've made my best effort at avoiding trigger factors and placing myself in a favorable position in the FM balance by managing susceptibility.   Despite my best efforts at controlling trigger and susceptibility factors I'm still prone to fall into FM symptoms. It's rarer these days now that I'm aware of so many of the factors, but it's still a part of my life.

I've come to realize that I can anticipate the approach of a full-blown FM event by some hours if I pay strict attention to certain warning signs and precursor symptoms. These initial stages are critical because it is much easier to halt the progression of symptoms here than it is once the full FM event begins. Experience has proven to me that taking immediate action with the onset of the earliest symptoms can often head off what would otherwise be a full FM event.

Admittedly I don't have the benefit of a control – I can't be certain that my early corrective actions are the reason my symptoms abate. On the other hand, I have the benefit of many iterations of intervention against what appear to be oncoming pain cycles that allow me to assess the results of taking these compensating actions and the results of not doing so. It's not a particularly efficient process but over time it has been an effective one.

While there's a short list of interventions at this stage it's an especially important list. I'm convinced these have on many occasions halted the progression of symptoms into what would have been an active FM event.

Figure 4: Managing an Approaching Event

- Pay attention to precursor symptoms.
- Begin using TENS - Transcutaneous electrical nerve stimulation.

"Precursor" symptoms

Success at this stage requires being aware of my physical state, one of the compensation techniques I mentioned earlier. One aspect of this is maintaining awareness in general – paying attention to how I feel at any given time (more accurately, paying attention periodically throughout the day). It's also important to know what the early symptoms of an FM event feel like, what I'm calling the "Precursor symptoms", because they are different from those of the FM event.

When I feel an FM event coming on it generally starts with the same indications: a subtle tightening of muscles in my head, neck, shoulders, and/or back. There's no real pain at this point, just a certain tight feeling that's not present when I'm otherwise well. It's easy to miss this stage completely unless you are looking for it, but it's an important one - this is the time to start compensating for what might otherwise be a further deepening of symptoms.

This tightening of muscles isn't always in the same location but generally is present in some combination of muscles that attach my shoulder and spine at a location high on my back. It often makes its presence known first in the Trapezius muscle where it runs parallel to the floor, between its shoulder attachment and my spine.

By tightening I mean what feels like a tensing of the muscles involved – and the relative inability to relax them to a normal state. If it's particularly strong (and it isn't always like this) it may feel like a low-level pins and needles sensation that won't go away easily.

Illustration 1: Trapezius Spasm Points

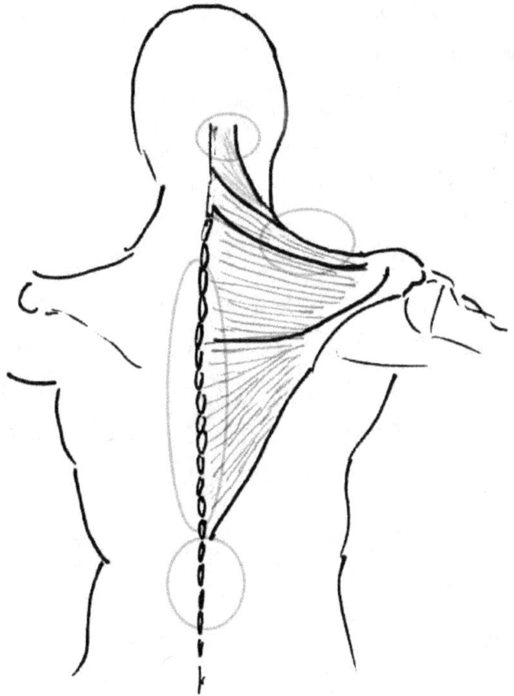

The circles in illustration 1 – a rear view of our human anatomy from the waist to head and shoulders - show where in my back I experience muscles in spasm, as well as the early symptoms of tightening and pressure. They seem related to various sectors of the Trapezius muscle or its attachment points and they most often occur on my right side.

If I sense this tightening early enough, I can confirm it by pressing on the affected muscle which will be painful and noticeably firm, as if it were locked in spasm. Without that pressure I might not experience classic pain but instead – at least at this stage – only the tightening sensation.

There is another, rarer pattern of symptom development that I see on occasion that doesn't follow the muscle-tightening route, at least not in the beginning. It's more of a pressure in my shoulders and back, almost as if a heavy weight were being pressed down on them from above. It's a strange sensation, as if I were carrying a weighted blanket over one side of my shoulders and neck resulting in a broad pressure, not unlike carrying a backpack or shoulder bag but more widely spread. If it's particularly strong it can even extend into the muscles of my face. This pressure-like pattern will eventually transition into traditional muscle tightening unless I can successfully head it off with one or more compensations.

If the FM symptoms continue to progress, they will advance into other shoulder and neck muscles, but often in the earliest stages only the topmost edge of the Trapezius is involved. This specific location is often a bellwether for me – if that spot begins to tighten, and then throb, I know I'm on my way to further FM symptoms. It's an early sign that I need to begin countermeasures.

A third pattern stems from strong trigger factors such as yellow dye or cured meats. Once the initial prolog period is over and the pain starts these can bypass the early symptoms entirely and progress directly into a full-blown FM event very quickly (within minutes or perhaps two hours, at most). Now that I have most of these strong factors under control that's a rare occurrence, I almost always get advance notice by the presence of this subtle tightening.

I don't accept the progression of symptoms from early signs to an FM event as inevitable – I know from experience that it can often be headed off at this point unless it has the force of one of the strong trigger factors behind it. Even then it can often be delayed until I'm in a better position to apply the serious countermeasures - those that are more disruptive to normal activities.

These early symptoms are clearer today than when I was in the depths of FM pain, before making the progress I've made over the past 15 years. I now see that I was in pain most of the time during those dark years, so much so that precursor symptoms had less meaning. There was no state of true "wellness" from which to descend into pain, I was constantly experiencing precursor symptoms – they were as good as things got for me. It took the improvements that came from better sleep and control over some of my stronger factors before this stage became evident. It also required a greater awareness of my physical state before I could sense them early enough to make a difference. It's one thing to realize there were precursor symptoms after an FM event begins, but quite another to recognize them before it arrives. This is the payback from mindfulness.

Identifying precursor symptoms is important because it can lead to earlier interventions with posture and rest, as well as the start of TENS use, where earlier is better.

TENS - Transcutaneous electrical nerve stimulation

This may sound frightening at first – but it's been a revolutionary technique for me, often warding off pain completely or reducing it to a low enough level so I can continue with daily life and not experience the disruption of a full FM event.

At its most basic - a TENS unit passes a low-level electric current through your skin, causing a tingling sensation and perhaps muscle movement – "twitching" in the underlying muscles. You can adjust its intensity and rhythm and choose where to apply it.

One theory suggests a TENS unit stimulates the same pathways in your nerves that pain is taking, but that this stimulation takes precedence over pain signals, hence blocking or reducing their impact. Others suggest that brain chemicals are changed in ways that have the same effect – pain reduction.

There are two types of TENS units, "conventional TENS" (the one that I use) passes current through pads stuck to your skin. "AL-TENS", acupuncture-like TENS, passes current into needles inserted into your skin. I selected the conventional "pad" type. I'll identify it in the Resources section.

I've had a lot of success using a conventional TENS unit at the first sign of FM pain to greatly reduce or even block its impact entirely. I'm using one as I stand here editing this section, having been exposed to road salt when doing errands yesterday afternoon. The pain started around breakfast, about 14 hours after I was exposed, despite taking the compensations I describe under the road salt trigger section.

I've tried numerous pad placement and current adjustments, finally settling on a starting pattern that seems to work best for me: I place two pads from one circuit on my lower back – under where my belt comes – and adjust the current style to one that varies in intensity and which pulses. This covers pain that is present in a wide area throughout my lower back up to my neck and face.

Though I've had some success applying stimulation to the actual painful areas on my back and shoulders, this lower back placement works best for me, especially as the first place I start when I begin using the TENS unit. I'm not generally experiencing pain at the pad locations – I suspect this blocks nerve pathways shared by other areas, or in the brain – at least that's how I look at it. Regardless, it took time to find the right combination of location, "program" (pulsation pattern and frequency), and intensity. Directly stimulating the areas of greatest pain was far less effective.

One caveat – this doesn't seem to work as well for the strongest triggers – yellow 6 and nitrate/nitrites. These build up to more serious pain regardless of how I use the TENS unit, although their overall severity seems to be reduced significantly. In short, it works less well for these triggers, but it helps.

Relief can take time to achieve, I usually start on a lower intensity setting and settle into a good chair or into bed to see what happens over the next half hour. It may require an increase in intensity and could take several hours to see full relief. A particularly intense FM event could require using the TENS unit off and on all day long and may not provide full relief.

With a low level of pain, I might continue with daily activities, snaking the lead wire up to a pocket where I can keep the TENS unit itself (I use a single set of pads, not both available channels).

The directions say "don't use while sleeping" though I find it helps me to use it "in bed" – helping me to return to sleep when I am wakened by an oncoming FM event. If I'm in pain I'm not sleeping. Using the TENS unit there brings me to a state where I can return to sleep. It runs on a timer so it turns off automatically.

As with any medical device – read and understand the directions and warning – there are places you shouldn't use the pads and people with conditions that preclude them entirely (for example, those with pacemakers).

Illustration 2: TENS Pad Placement

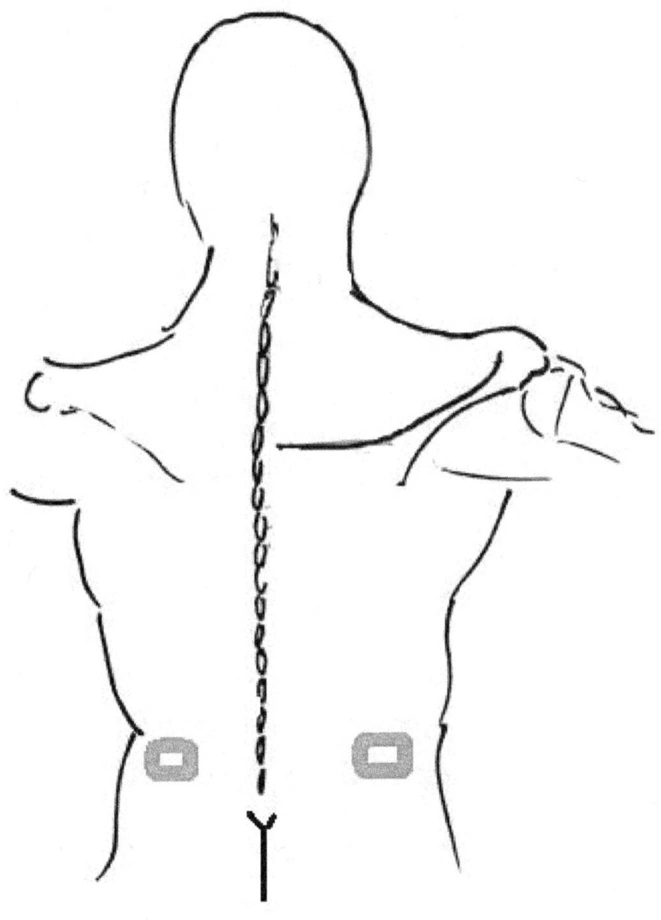

In the past, without the TENS unit, I would progress more easily through the phases of pain to a full-blown FM event. I would then need to retire from daily life – finding a dark, quiet place, lying on an exercise mat on the floor for support, covered by a quilt to stay warm, stretching taut muscles – while waiting for the pain to first peak and then subside over the next 8 to 24 hours, simply enduring it. The TENS unit can dramatically reduce the impact of an oncoming FM event (if not stopping it in its tracks) and preclude the need for more dramatic steps.

Recovery is faster and easier as well – eventually the pain (the pain that makes it through the TENS technique) subsides. Rather than feeling as if I've recovered from a bout of influenza, the pain disappears, and I return quickly to normal.

Recovering from an FM event:

Eventually, on FM's schedule, the pain subsides, and I return to normal. That's the time to begin evaluating what might have gone wrong with my carefully laid FM management plans. This includes asking the questions:

- What might have contributed to the FM event?

- Have I uncovered a new trigger or am I relatively sure which known trigger was involved?
- Have I found a new food I need to avoid, a new product containing yellow dye or another known trigger?
- Have I found a new compensation technique in my attempts to deal with the pain?

Regardless of my success in identifying the factor or factors involved, it's time to move on and try to return to a normal routine – to put the pain behind me and begin again as if it had never occurred.

Caffeine

Caffeine deserves a closer look here in the compensations chapter as it can be either a compounding factor or compensation, depending on how and when it's used.

I've previously considered it a compounding factor as it turns up in several OTC pain relievers where it can simply make matters worse should I take them in the evening – when I'm most in need of relief. Too much caffeine in beverages can also interfere with my sleep, becoming a trigger all on its own.

And yet caffeine in the morning can contribute to the relief of FM symptoms – so it's a two-edged sword. So long as I manage the amount and timing of caffeine, I'm able to continue to enjoy coffee and tea daily. In fact, it can help to bring me out of the release stage of an FM event.

Chapter Summary

- Compensations are actions taken to defer, avoid, or reduce FM pain.
- Avoidance is ideal - no exposure equals no pain.
- OTC Pain relievers have been of no help to me, they simply have no effect. Some actually contain known triggers of pain.
- Actions before exposure:
    - getting proper sleep
    - avoiding triggers
    - maintaining FM situational awareness
    - managing stress
    - getting exercise, maintaining posture
- Actions after exposure:
    - watching for the start of symptoms (precursor symptoms)
    - using TENS (Transcutaneous electrical nerve stimulation)
- Caffeine is fine so long as it's managed carefully – it doesn't belong in the afternoon/evening but can help encourage the release stage of an FM event.

Approach

So where does this lead us? How do you use what I've learned to avoid FM pain and major events?

In "Coping with Fibromyalgia" I devoted an entire chapter to "approach" – describing how I went about finding and managing the sources of FM pain I knew at the time. If the triggers I found using those methods are not shared with other fibromyalgia sufferers - or if there are significantly more triggers out there that I simply haven't found - then this original detailed approach to rooting out chemical triggers is called for. You may need to find your own unique triggers and techniques for avoiding them. If these triggers are unique to me or you are sensitive to something I'm not exposed to you'll need to read the Approach chapter in "Coping with Fibromyalgia" for a more detailed view of how I found these triggers in myself.

But if, as I suspect, these triggers are not unique to me – if they have the same effect on others as they have on me - then we can take some shortcuts. Certainly, that's the best place to start. Begin by finding and limiting your exposure to the triggers I've listed above and see if they have an effect in reducing pain events. Pay attention to the compounding factors I've found to be related to my overall FM experience – especially sleep. And finally, try the compensations I've found to help in dealing with exposure when avoidance isn't practical.

Know also that it took time for me to pull out of the pain cycles I had fallen into even as I reduced exposure to these triggers. It didn't happen overnight and, while it was in part driven by the avoidance of triggers that developed over time, I continue to practice all three techniques: avoidance, compensation and attention to the factors that compound the pain.

The original, detailed approach outlined in "Coping with Fibromyalgia" continues to describe how I view food and my environment so I'll summarize it here but refer you back to that detailed account should you relate to what I've described in the earlier chapters in this book.

Three erroneous assumptions

- Our food supply is "safe" – I can't be harmed by what I eat.
- Relief from pain can only come in the form of medication.
- Relief from pain can come without changes in my behavior.

It was necessary to overcome these basic beliefs to uncover the sources of my FM pain and begin to address them successfully.

The identification of clear chemical triggers for FM pain has led me to a new way of thinking and acting. It's an approach to coping that crosses the categories I've outlined earlier in this book. While it's easier to explain them individually in the way they're organized in earlier chapters, that is not how I think about them each day. My actions are arranged around exposure to a trigger – the actions I take before and after pain arrives. I can sometimes anticipate pain, other times not. I've described these in detail in earlier chapters but let me summarize them here in a new context, one of thought and behavior.

Illustration 3: Hierarchy of Coping Actions

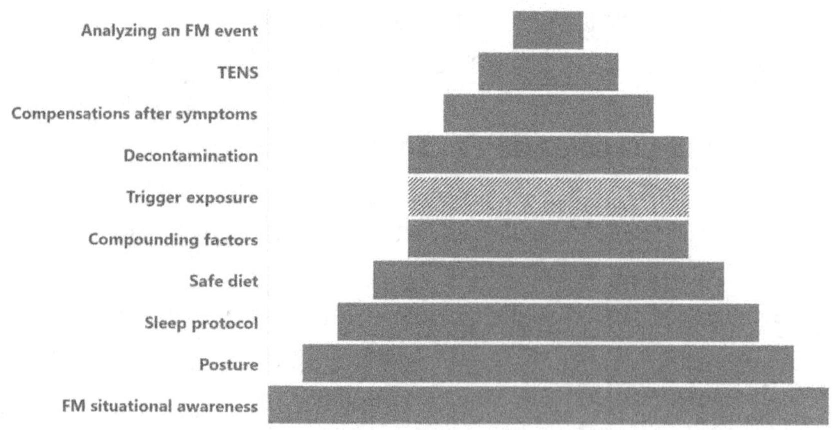

FM situational awareness

I'm now describing my overall FM balance as "maintaining FM situational awareness" - paying attention to my physical state, recognizing the onset of FM symptoms, and beginning to ask, "how did this happen". It really means always keeping the hierarchy of coping actions in mind, changing daily behavior to avoid exposure and, when that fails, asking what the initiating trigger could be, where did exposure originate?

Posture

Posture is always in the back of my mind, wherever I am and whatever I'm doing. It may or may not be directly related to FM pain, but it certainly can be a source of discomfort that I don't want to add to the equation.

Compounding factors and sleep protocol

To be honest, I usually identify these after I begin feeling pain – thinking back to what might be leading me here. But I also give some thought to "susceptibility", for example, around the time barometric pressure might drop (as in a hurricane). I also pay close attention to my sleep patterns and attempt to recover whenever I sleep poorly. Maintaining adequate quality sleep is core to my success in FM management and is always on my mind.

Finding a safe diet

This begins by **always** reading food labels. As imperfect as this is I still focus on the ingredient list before I try any new food. In the early days it was needed to identify any new ingredient that might be causing issues, but it's now needed to identify those that contain one of my trigger chemicals.

I began this effort rather narrowly, just reading (and believing) the ingredient lists on food. Today this is only a starting point, I pay strict attention to any new food or meal ingredients, watching carefully to see if I can tolerate it - whether home cooked or purchased and regardless of what's shown in the ingredients.

I view food very differently than I did in the past, viewing every meal as containing a potential FM trigger if there's anything "new" about it. I take chances with new things, but I pay attention when I do. I'm more careful about where I buy food and from where it's sourced. I pay attention to the components of prepared foods, avoiding the things I now know I can't tolerate.

One core behavior I've developed over the years has been to identify, and stick to, a "safe" core diet. I've identified a specific list of foods and drinks that I can trust will not trigger my FM symptoms – that truly do not contain any of the trigger compounds I've come to know are unsafe for me.

This wasn't as easy as it sounds, both in identifying these foods and limiting my intake to them. While it's not exactly a hermit's fare, every variation from it presents a risk. It's challenging during the holidays, when travelling, or when dining out.

I find myself straying from this core on occasion, especially after I've been free from FM symptoms for several weeks or months. I forget the need for discipline – but I'm quickly brought back into line should I happen onto a new, unsafe source.

Any new food not on my "safe list" is an experiment in sensitivity and a test of its ingredient list. Test failures are not rare.

Trigger exposure

This can come unexpectedly, such as with a new food item, or I may know it's coming, as with road salt. Either way, it's the deciding event between preparing for and reacting to an FM pain event.

Decontamination

Removing all traces of road salt is a major step I've learned to take as soon after exposure as possible. It's driven by the degree of exposure, both in terms of time and dosage, so to speak.

TENS and compensations after symptoms

TENS – transcutaneous electrical nerve stimulation – isn't the first step I take after pain begins, but it's now an important one to consider. It's not always needed but can be a major step that can either halt the progression of pain toward a full-blown event or reduce its impact substantially. I wish this had been available to me forty years ago.

Analyzing an FM event

Once the pain of an event has begun to subside, I begin to ask, "how did this happen". At times (as with road salt) I know when exposure occurred, but if not, I need to ask where exposure occurred.

It's not easy to do this during a pain event, nor is it easy when the pain finally abates to think back 24 hours or more to identify what you may have been exposed to. Yet it's been key to my success in finding the sources of my FM pain.

Each FM pain event is a "natural experiment" in our response to the environment which for me means "what chemicals I've been exposed to". It's less open ended for me these days having identified the major sources of pain, but I'm always on the lookout for something I may have missed. I'm especially careful with chocolate – it's currently the riskiest new food I would encounter.

Final recommendations

If you can relate to what I've described here and suffer from similarly unexplained chronic pain, **try identifying and reducing your exposure to the triggers I've identified above.** I'd suggest starting with yellow 6 and the nitrates/nitrites in preserved meats as they are such strong triggers. Controlling them could – if you share these sensitivities – show results quickly.

Road salt is much harder to control, but it's possible by taking the decontamination steps I outline in the Triggers chapter. But without controlling exposure to road salt, you can expect to reach and maintain a certain ongoing level of pain during the winter season until spring/summer rains wash away the contaminant.

Admittedly, I may be unique in my sensitivity to widely used chemicals and the pain of other FM sufferers may originate in completely different circumstances. But this approach has worked well for me, I'm able to go for prolonged periods without a major FM event and can better anticipate and understand the pain I'm not able to evade.

I've previously described this as a balance – the "Fibromyalgia Balance". It's akin to riding a bicycle. You're navigating between a safe diet without chemical exposures versus pain, over a path that can be smoothed by healthy practices. A mistake that veers you toward pain leaves you with only a few, unsatisfactory pain-reduction options. Repeated missteps raise the bar into chronic pain and all the other unwanted FM symptoms.

Finally, make pain relief the last tool in your war chest, not the first.

Chapter Summary

- Three erroneous assumptions:
  - our food supply is safe.
  - medication can relieve pain.
  - pain relief can come without behavioral change.
- Analyze every FM event for root causes.
- Think about FM in terms of pre- and post-pain coping actions.
- Look at every FM event as a "natural experiment" in chemical exposure.
- Always read food labels, particularly on any new food.
- Find a "safe diet", a core set of food items that are not related to your FM symptoms.
- Reduce your exposure to the triggers listed here and watch for reduced FM symptoms.
- Consider all this a balancing act between avoiding environmental exposures versus living in pain.
- Make pain relief the last tool in your war chest against FM.

Chemical Safety

This is where I'd like to include a chapter on chemical safety – laying out the nature of the chemicals I'm susceptible to and how they are being managed.

Unfortunately, they're not being managed - it's extremely difficult to find information on the nature and effects of the substances I've identified as triggers for pain – even those being directly added to our food. What little information I found over the past two years as I researched for this book is no longer available. Several studies into the effects of road salt on the environment (albeit with little regard for its effects on humans) are no longer found on their original websites. Formal research into the effects of road salt largely ignores the added ingredients, focusing instead on the effects of salt on the environment.

Chemical safety data sheets required by U.S. regulations have recently been scrubbed of any information remotely detrimental to their sales and use. Written by the manufacturers and copyrighted to prevent widespread access, chemicals once described in rather frightening terms are now largely shown with "no data available" for important categories of reporting.

The three strongest triggers – yellow 6, sodium nitrate/nitrite, and sodium ferrocyanide – when you can find a Safety Data Sheet - often suggest wearing gloves and eye protection when handling. Bon appetite.

I suspect from long experience with chocolate that ingredient lists on products are not all-inclusive. Unexpected items make it into the mix. The variety of names that can be used to refer to these chemicals is startling. Even if something is listed in the "ingredients" who really knows what that is?

PubChem, the reference facility maintained by the National Institute of Health, National Library of Medicine is an interesting reference for the base substances I've identified here as causing my FM pain, but there's no easy cross reference between the various chemicals listed there and where we are exposed to them.

Reviewing cured meats on numerous retailer pages shows an interesting pattern: the ingredients in "uncured" meats are often readily available in images of the back side of the product or listed in the description. The ingredients in "cured" meats are often unavailable, with no image of the "ingredients" side of the package and no listing in the description.

What this all means to me is that, like so many things, we're on our own in our navigation through food and the environment.

This topic deserves its own book – from someone closer to the systems, technology, and biology than I am.

Conclusions

I am acutely sensitive to several commonly used substances in the environment, I'm calling them triggers:

- **Sodium ferrocyanide** – an additive in bulk road salt commonly used in the northern United States, often under the name yellow prussiate of soda.
- **Sodium Nitrate/Sodium Nitrite** - the food additives often used to cure meat in the U.S.
- **Yellow 6** – a.k.a. Sunset Yellow FCA - a food dye approved by the FDA for use in coloring a variety of products, including chocolate.
- **Numerous modern home products as well as several organic food additives** – including bergamot, cloves, and annatto.

These triggers are directly related to the chronic pain I experience as a fibromyalgia sufferer. While "it's the dose that makes the poison", I regularly see symptoms at the levels of exposure I'm afforded in daily life. Those symptoms can be disabling, involving pain equivalent to a multi-day long migraine.

I suspect there are other chemicals that have the same negative effects on me, but I haven't had the repeated exposures needed to clearly identify them.

I found these triggers heuristically – through basic trial and error. It took many years of attention to isolate the effects of these common substances to which I was regularly being exposed.

On the one hand, I find it hard to believe I'm alone in my sensitivity to various common chemicals and ingredients and that others aren't reporting success in mitigating fibromyalgia by controlling their exposure to them. On the other hand, I can understand how this could come about. Here are some reasons they are not easy to discover:

- These trigger substances are widely used – commonly occurring in our food and environment.
- As such, it's easy to be exposed to multiple triggers at once, complicating any effort to identify what's at fault.
- There is an hours-long delay between exposure to a trigger and the onset of symptoms, further complicating discovery.
- As a consumer, it is difficult to identify the ingredients we're being exposed to in our food and the environment.

- We all face challenges in identifying the nature and safety of chemicals in use – both in the workforce and in our food and environment.
- There is an assumption of safety behind many of our long-used industrial age chemicals, I see little evidence they've been carefully vetted for safety.
- There are "compounding factors" which, though they do not directly cause pain, are related to the degree and speed at which the triggers work.
- There are other sources for pain unrelated to the FM triggers I've listed here.

These factors all work against exposing these substances as "irritants". When you also consider the lack of objective measures for pain it's no wonder we haven't identified these as 'irritants". Their individual impacts are lost in a soup of overlapping exposures, subjective measures, misinformation about food ingredients, and outdated industrial age assumptions.

Two "non-chemical" triggers – lack of sleep and recovery from influenza – further complicate the identification of the primary chemical triggers.

And finally, if all this wasn't bad enough, the underlying pain these triggers cause can become a "new normal", the baseline against which normality is measured. It's necessary to see substantial success in eliminating the underlying pain – to reach a plateau of relief – before the individual triggers begin to show themselves clearly.

These findings also suffer from the observation that "extraordinary claims require extraordinary evidence". It would be disruptive to remove these substances from our environment, and powerful interests are lined up against doing so. The few times I've seen researchers approach the effects of road salt additives their findings have been withdrawn from view. I would observe that chemical "safety data sheets" have been scrubbed of any possible negative effects for the people who use chemicals daily. I can only describe what I find to be effective for me and hope it adds to the accumulated knowledge developing as we pay stricter attention to ourselves and the environment we live in.

And to be fair, I'm not aware of any other person who can confirm my observations. These triggers may be limited to me. Sensitivity could span more chemicals than I've uncovered and/or be derived dynamically. They might even be unique to each individual. But I find this hard to believe – that I am unique in this sensitivity. These chemicals are simply too common to avoid and thus individually identify as irritants. Finally, there are too many others experiencing unexplained, chronic pain for each person's affliction to be unique.

While avoidance is the simplest answer to all this – it's not possible with some triggers and not practical with others. Road salt is the worst offender – I'm exposed for 6 months each year, traveling on public roads is part of life in the rural area in which I live. I suspect yellow 6 is being used at some point in the chocolate trade and doesn't make it to the ingredient list. Chocolate is almost ubiquitous in food; I'm forced to experiment on myself with every new brand/variety/use. Ingredients that include nitrates/nitrites are being hidden by some retailers – it can take a concerted effort to uncover them.

I can find relief by compensating in several ways, but these techniques impose restrictions on my life that I would rather avoid. At best these trigger substances should be removed from use; at the very least, we should be given the opportunity to avoid them.

If I'm not alone in this sensitivity, how many others can be spared chronic pain and the well-known risks inherent in its treatment?

If I'm not alone in this, then we need to take the following actions:

- A replacement for sodium ferrocyanide must be found for the manufacture of road salt. It's not practical to avoid it, something less irritating needs to be used in its place. It may be contributing to the increasing incidence of chronic pain being seen in the US in recent years.
- Ideally, the nitrate/nitrite compounds used to cure meat and the food dye yellow 6 would be banned. At the very least, open and accurate reporting must be required at all points in the sales process.
- Manufacturers must disclose all the ingredients in food and retailers (particularly web retailers) must fully disclose product ingredient lists.
- We need to research the use of yellow 6 in chocolate. If it's not simply banned, it should be subject to the above reporting requirements and be exposed on the ingredients list of all products that contain it.
- Fibromyalgia sufferers and researchers need to consider the possibility of chemical triggers for pain – including the substances I've identified and others I haven't encountered or that may be unique to individuals.

We need to view pain as a significant social and economic burden akin to an epidemic.

169

Resources

American Heart Association
http://www.americanheart.org

"The Art of Body Maintenance: Winner's Guide to Pain Relief"
by Hal Blatman and Brad Ekvall. Danua Press
2002, 2006

As You Sow, Toxins in Chocolate testing
https://www.asyousow.org/environmental-health/toxic-enforcement/toxic-chocolate#chocolate-tables

Chemical Abstracts Service
https://www.cas.org/

"The Chemistry of Road Salt And How It Works",
American Chemistry Council LabNotes (notably omitting any mention of additives)
https://www.americanchemistry.com/chemistry-in-america/news-trends/blog-post/2018/the-chemistry-of-road-salt-and-how-it-works

Devin Starlanyl (numerous books)

Dr. Andrew Weil
http://www.drweil.com/

"Facts and myths pertaining to fibromyalgia",
Winfried Häuser, MD*, Mary-Ann Fitzcharles,
MD, NIH National Library of Medicine, Dialogues
in Clinical Neuroscience, March 2018.
https://www.ncbi.nlm.nih.gov/pmc/articles/PM
C6016048/

"Food: The Chemistry of Its Components", Tom
Coultate, Royal Society of Chemistry, 2009
https://www.google.com/books/edition/Food/K
F2A8Cz7B-cC?hl=en&gbpv=1

Healthy Sleep site at Harvard
http://healthysleep.med.harvard.edu/

iReliev TENS unit (available from Disk's Sporting
Goods, Amazon and the iRelieve website)
https://ireliev.com/product/tens-ems-combo-
muscle-stimulator/

"Mayo Clinic Guide to Fibromyalgia"
By Andy Abril and Barbara K. Bruce Oct 1, 2020

Mayo Clinic Fibromyalgia pages for December 4,
2010, from the Internet Archive "Wayback
Machine"

https://web.archive.org/web/20101203225234/http://www.mayoclinic.com/health/fibromyalgia/DS00079

Mayo Clinic Fibromyalgia page - current
https://www.mayoclinic.org/diseases-conditions/fibromyalgia/symptoms-causes/syc-20354780

National Fibromyalgia Association
http://www.fmaware.org

National Institute of Arthritis and Musculoskeletal and Skin Diseases
http://www.niams.nih.gov/Health_Info/Fibromyalgia/

National Institutes of Health
https://www.niams.nih.gov/health-topics/fibromyalgia/advanced#tab-overview

National Library of Medicine – PubChem database
https://pubchem.ncbi.nlm.nih.gov/

National Center for Biotechnology Information (2023). PubChem Compound Summary for CID 26129, Sodium ferrocyanide. Retrieved February 1, 2023
from https://pubchem.ncbi.nlm.nih.gov/compound/Sodium-ferrocyanide

National Center for Biotechnology Information
(2023). PubChem Compound Summary for CID
24268, Sodium Nitrate. Retrieved February 1,
2023
from https://pubchem.ncbi.nlm.nih.gov/compo
und/Sodium-Nitrate

National Center for Biotechnology Information
(2023). PubChem Compound Summary for CID
23668193, Sodium nitrite. Retrieved February 1,
2023
from https://pubchem.ncbi.nlm.nih.gov/compo
und/Sodium-nitrite

NeilMed Sinus Rinse – nasal lavage kit
https://shop.neilmed.com/collections/sinus-
rinse

"Pain Trends Among American Adults, 2002–
2018: Patterns, Disparities, and Correlates",
Demography, Duke University Press, April 1, 2021
https://read.dukeupress.edu/demography/articl
e/58/2/711/168526/Pain-Trends-Among-
American-Adults-2002-2018

"Posture Affects Standing, and Not Just the Physical Kind", Jane E. Brody, The New York Times, December 28, 2015
https://archive.nytimes.com/well.blogs.nytimes.com/2015/12/28/posture-affects-standing-and-not-just-the-physical-kind/?searchResultPosition=1

"Potential Water-Quality Effects from Iron Cyanide Anticaking Agents in Road Salt", Paschka et.al, Water Environment Research Sep-Oct 1999.
https://www.jstor.org/stable/25045306

"Risk Management Strategy for Road Salts", Environment Canada, archived from October 2003
https://web.archive.org/web/20040301045226/http://www.ec.gc.ca/nopp/roadsalt/reports/en/rms.cfm

Schmidt Sting Pain Index
https://en.wikipedia.org/wiki/Schmidt_sting_pain_index

Thich Nhat Hanh
http://en.wikipedia.org/wiki/Thich_Nhat_Hanh

"Trying the Feldenkrais Method for Chronic Pain", Jane E. Brody, New York Times, October 30, 2017
https://www.nytimes.com/2017/10/30/well/trying-the-feldenkrais-method-for-chronic-pain.html

Wikipedia entry: Curing (food preservation)
https://en.wikipedia.org/wiki/Curing_(food_preservation)

Wikipedia entry: Fibromyalgia
http://en.wikipedia.org/wiki/Fibromyalgia

Wikipedia entry: Sodium ferrocyanide
https://en.wikipedia.org/wiki/Sodium_ferrocyanide

Wikipedia entry: Sodium Nitrate
https://en.wikipedia.org/wiki/Sodium_nitrate

Wikipedia entry: Sodium Nitrite
https://en.wikipedia.org/wiki/Sodium_nitrite

Wikipedia entry: Sunset yellow FCF
https://en.wikipedia.org/wiki/Sunset_yellow_FCF

Yellow Prussiate of Soda admixture to create Road Salt (Cargill Corp.)
https://www.cargill.com/industrial/winter-road-maintenance/deicers

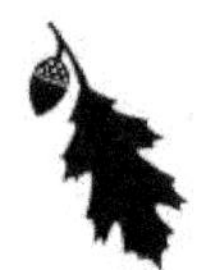